Every Last Breat

# Every Last Breath

*A Memoir of Two Illnesses*

Joanne Jacobson

THE UNIVERSITY OF UTAH PRESS
*Salt Lake City*

The Defiance House Man colophon is a registered trademark
of The University of Utah Press. It is based on a four-foot-tall
Ancient Puebloan pictograph (late PIII) near Glen Canyon, Utah.

Library of Congress Cataloging-in-Publication Data
Names: Jacobson, Joanne, 1952– author.
Title: Every last breath / Joanne Jacobson.
Description: Salt Lake City : The University of Utah Press, [2020]
Identifiers: LCCN 2020014572 (print) | LCCN 2020014573 (ebook) |
ISBN 9781647690014 (paperback) | ISBN 9781647690021 (ebook)
Subjects: LCSH: Critically ill—Medical care—Psychological aspects. |
  Terminally ill—Psychology. | Blood—Diseases. | Respiratory
  organs—Diseases.
Classification: LCC R726.8 .J33 2020  (print) | LCC R726.8  (ebook) |
DDC 616.02/9—dc23
LC record available at https://lccn.loc.gov/2020014572
LC ebook record available at https://lccn.loc.gov/2020014573

"Every Last Breath" appeared in *Fourth Genre*.
  Copyright © 2011 by Michigan State University.
"Economy" appeared in *Atrium: The Report of the Northwestern Medical
  Humanities and Bioethics Program* (2011).
"Goodbye and Goodbye" appeared in *Great River Review* (2011).
"In the Year of Masking Tape" appeared in *Florida Review* (2015).
"Mirror Writing" appeared in *Tampa Review* (2016).
"Written in Blood" appeared in *Southwest Review* (2016).
"If My Disease Were an Animal" appeared, under a slightly different
  title, in *Gulf Coast Online* (2016).
"Dead Reckoning" appeared in *Seneca Review* (2013).
"My Mother, Gardening" appeared in *New England Review* (2013).
"Thoreau's Body" appeared, in a revised version, in *Bellevue Literary
  Review* (2018).

Errata and further information on this and other titles available online
at UofUpress.com.

Printed and bound in the United States of America.

for Ellen

# Contents

My mother lies lit in the night, asleep beside her bedroom lamp, a book splayed across her chest. For a moment I worry once again that she's stopped breathing, but now I see the slight rise of lace at the opened neck of her worn flannel nightgown, the wrinkled skin around the little O of her mouth tightening and releasing. Her television is blaring at hard-of-hearing pitch and flashing images of Ted Kennedy's funeral from this morning: Kennedy children and grandchildren arriving in the rain, their faces as familiar as ever after two generations of public deaths; George W. Bush and Bill Clinton entering the modest neighborhood church and taking their places in the pew of former presidents; the cutaway images of Ted sailing off Hyannis, happy in his windbreaker, his thick white hair flying in the wind. He was seventy-seven years old, seven years younger than my mother, when he died three days ago.

I turn off the TV and slip into the kitchen, flipping switches as I go. When I open the refrigerator, halved tomatoes and onions and peppers are light-flooded, hooded in Saran Wrap, rocking slightly as the heavy door swings to one side. Shreds of jam and mayo cling to the sides of jars in my mother's refrigerator, enough for one morning's slice of toast or one more tuna salad sandwich. A single slice of Swiss cheese is laid out on a glass shelf between sheets of wax paper.

Contemplating her cabinets for the thousandth time, I can feel her hoarded stuff pressing from the inside: the plastic husks of *margarine tubs and old Cool Whip containers stacked compression-tight; the jumble of bamboo cocktail skewers and the colored Styrofoam jackets for hot coffee and tea, ready for a barbecue or a picnic; a rubber-banded stack of party napkins. OK, I think, facing the stained dish towel still hanging after my mother returned the new set that my sister and I bought for Mother's Day,* OK, this is her deal with the universe: nothing released too soon into the careless spin of things.

# Every Last Breath

What lives, breathes. Listen.

It's not my strokes that I hear when I swim, muscles working through choppy water, slaps and kicks breaking the surface, but the sound of my own breath: spitting, animal hunger for air. Open-mouthed, needing, I rise, sucking from what's just above the wet. Every heaving breath—the living body knows—could be the last.

In the high quiet above the earth, migrating birds can hear life itself, the beat of wings and of breath taking them to where there is food and where they can breed, the cycle beginning again every year. They sweep the sky in flocks so thick that they shadow the land below. The monarch butterfly—one-fifth of an ounce!—finds its way the length of the continent north to south, fueled by air, sweet air setting wafer wings in vibration.

From every room in her apartment, I can hear my mother's breath. The steady hiss of force—not her own—drawing from tubes and canisters in the interstices of television sound. Clear plastic is clipped in her nostrils, crossing her face; tubing curls and uncurls in her wake. She turns and whips the knotting line behind her, untangling and clearing, making her careful way from the hall to the kitchen. She is feeding on oxygen.

Her breath used to quicken in the summer sun as she inhaled in even gulps between sets of tennis, balancing casually on the handle of her racquet. What required air she could easily do: take the green lawn with the mower in long, circling rows, leaving stacked clippings drying behind her in the heat; rake the heavy leaves to the curb at the chill, wet end of autumn; paint the kitchen walls; unload groceries from the car, lug bags up the sidewalk from the garage, jam open the screen door with one crooked arm while she balanced a sack of canned soup and frozen vegetables and a half-gallon of skim milk with the other. She'd wait for my little sister to climb the back steps one by one and then steer her through the spring door that strained against her own back: *Scoot!*

My mother's oxygen is delivered now, pumped into a green drum half my height in the front hall. She fills a canister when she leaves the house and straps it to her back, counting the minutes. Breathing has become work. She crosses slowly to the window every morning, laying down a cord trail behind her bathrobe, and pours seed for the birds that wait at her feeder. In her little yard, cardinals and jays screech and flicker, bold red and blue above the ragged lawn. They dive and grab for what my mother gives them, recklessly leaving a cloud of discarded husks, squandering the fresh air.

*I remember waiting at railroad crossings with my mother on our way to visit my aunt and my cousins, the two of us drifting off together in the front seat of her Dodge Dart, the summer heat gathering around us, as hundreds of loaded boxcars and empty flatbeds clacked past. Sometimes we would count them, or count the minutes they took up as they went by. Wild grasses lined the tracks for miles, blurred in the strong sun, last remnants of the prairies that spanned the raw center of the continent before the steel plow buried them alive to carve out space for the world's growing wheat. We'd watch for the caboose, squinting into the light until it came into view and then finally lumbered along, headed for mysterious destinations painted on the rusted sides of the cars: Santa Fe; Burlington; Pennsylvania; Topeka. When the last faraway whistle reached us from the train's lengthening wake, we'd stir as if from a trance and take deep breaths, almost in unison, before my mother bent in the warm, stilled air to turn her key in the ignition and set us in motion again.*

# Economy

My mother can drive to the doctor or the grocery store, but she cannot drive at night or in snow. Probably she shouldn't be driving at all, but she won't agree to give up her independence.

My mother can go on every day, even when she feels tired or chilled or discouraged—dressing herself and taking medication for the arthritis in her hip and back and neck and for high blood pressure—but she cannot beat back completely the respiratory infections that keep recurring and turning into pneumonia, more serious each time.

My mother cannot leave her apartment without an oxygen canister, but she can breathe on her own wherever she goes if she sits in a chair or on a sofa.

My mother cannot hear the conversation at the dinner table if she doesn't wear her hearing aids, and she cannot follow what others are saying unless they speak slowly and loudly and are prepared to repeat. She cannot wear hearing aids when her oxygen apparatus is hooked over her ears.

My mother cannot bend down to tie her own shoes, but she can make vegetarian chopped liver and cream of broccoli soup, and she can bake raspberry squares from the recipe she's been using since I was a kid. She cannot always keep her grandchildren's birthdays straight, but she can still manage the old Scrabble strategies, coming up with seven-letter words and boosting her score by building across the board on the colored double-letter and triple-word squares.

My mother can go to my sister and brother-in-law's house and sit drinking seltzer under the grape arbor that they just built in their backyard, but she cannot stay outside if there's wind. And she cannot fly alone from Chicago again to spend the month of January in warm Phoenix with her lifelong friend Clarice.

My mother can watch the birds shift with the seasons through the picture window in her living room, but she cannot return to Costa Rica, where we were lucky enough to catch sight of the resplendent quetzal through a field telescope—
*Can a bird draped in green, thick and lush as ermine, be real?* we asked one another in wonder—or to Sanibel Island, where we watched flocks of anhingas and gulls jam the scarlet, low-hanging sunset sky.

My mother can have Thanksgiving dinner with my sister's in-laws, an hour's drive from her house, and she can spend Passover at her nephew's, a mile away. But she cannot catch all the words of the Four Questions chanted in the reedy, hesitant voice of the youngest at the seder table. And she cannot any longer travel to Minnesota for the weddings and birthdays and bar and bat mitzvahs of her nephews and nieces, or to lay flowers on the grave there where they buried her older sister thirty years ago.

My mother can never visit me in New York again.

My mother cannot understand why my sister and I don't use coupons at the grocery store; why her downstairs neighbor blocks the driveway when she parks, or her upstairs neighbor has so many packages delivered; why Americans are so short-sighted about the environment; or why her own twin sister hardly ever calls her yet continues to complain that my mother doesn't call *her*! But she understands that her daughters are worried. She knows that we're measuring the strength of her voice over the phone, that we're checking with one another about her, that we're not completely convinced that she's okay.

My mother can arrange to have her apartment redecorated, she can select paint colors for four rooms and she can order fabric for new floor-to-ceiling drapes, but she cannot ask her doctor the hard questions: Why doesn't your office return my phone calls? *Will I be able to go outside this winter?*

I can fly home when my mother ends up in the emergency room, straining for air, but I can't find the patience for the long process of recovery from pneumonia—for the labored three-minute walks from her hospital room to the nurses' station with which she must slowly start, even though only a week before she was pushing her own cart through the grocery store. I can help my mother sort her bills into piles, paid and unpaid, on the dining room table: her monthly condo fees and electricity and water and heat; the contributions that she makes to her synagogue and to agencies committed to rebuilding progressive politics in Israel and to combating hunger all over the world. But she won't let me show her a better way to organize the pills that she deposits each morning into a discolored plastic container top on her kitchen counter, where they roll around the rim.

How can it take so long for my mother to get ready to go outside? I try not to count the minutes as she showers and decides what to wear; as she pulls up her socks with the long shoehorn on which she depends because of her arthritis; as she puts on her plastic mask and inhales medicated mist; as she makes breakfast and eats it; as she puts all the dishes in the sink and she wipes her placemat; as she fills her oxygen tank and she grabs the stamped mail; as she braces for her first cautious breath of chill, hurting air. My mother is no longer strong enough to clean her apartment, and she claims that she doesn't have the time to look for help or the money to pay for it. I try to convince her otherwise—she has plenty of both!—first reassuring and then squabbling with her, until both of us are weary although nothing is settled; until it's hard to remember love.

# Goodbye and Goodbye

I

Goodbye, old clothes.

My sister and I are helping our mother pare down the contents of her closets and her eight-drawer wooden dresser—getting her ready to move to a retirement home. My mother works slowly, hanger by hanger, holding up the knit jackets and the soft wool sweaters that she wears to synagogue on Friday nights, unfolding the brightly colored scarves that we've been buying for her birthdays and for Mother's Day. We ask her to try them on for us, and she unpeels the flowered sweatshirt and the faded jeans that she wears every day around the apartment. I feel a ripple of shyness, but my mother doesn't bother to turn away. Anita and I see her eighty-five-year-old skin slipping in spots from her arms, and the varicose veins streaking blue up and down her legs. She no longer fills her bra completely.

Many of my mother's favorite clothes—the silk appliqué blazer, not even three years old, and the trench coat that we gave her—hang slack now. She seems to feel her smallness herself as she closes a row of buttons, and she looks down at her loosely swaddled body as she reads our faces. My mother gathers a bulky hand-knit sweater around her shoulders, and her voice fills with emotion: "I love wearing this one!" She lays out on her bed four red turtlenecks and three blue ones, then adds a stack of cardigans to the clothes that she intends to take with her. She has worn them all through years of bundling up for apple-picking and for the last backyard barbecue of the season, for walking along the lake on the first still-raw mornings of spring. I know that she is overwhelmed by the long task ahead, by the choosing and the packing and by the prospect of dressing for a new life among people whose faces and clothes she can't yet imagine.

Even for the snake—instinctual shedder of what's dear—the act of sloughing off can take a harsh toll. Beneath the molting layer the new skin is raw, unready for touch, freshly spun over beating heart. While it's shedding a snake's eyes grow cloudy, and its vision dims as it focuses on the hard work of shaking free: starting from the head, rubbing loose the leathery mouth and the nose; finishing by gulping water to slake the big thirst it's worked up. Only after it heaves its old skin aside can the snake fully resume seeing and breathing.

Wild, exhausting life, moving each passing year a little more slowly, each year a little more reluctant to let go of what sticks close, reluctant to release what matters.

**2**

"There's a revolution in the building!" my next-door neighbor in the Loire Valley town where I lived phoned one afternoon to let me know. My mother had hung her laundry out to dry on my apartment balcony. "Silly French people!" my mother said, not quietly, as she took down her wet jeans and stockings and I hovered self-consciously just inside. When I finally delivered my mother to the train station, I began waving goodbye as soon as the conductor set a stepstool for her near the tracks. I could see my mother through the windows, moving uncertainly through the car with her little suitcase, searching for the seat that I'd reserved for her. And before I could spot her getting settled, the train began to pull out toward Paris and the yellow letters on the side of each car—*S-N-C-F*—were passing me in a blur.

Months later, in cold rain, I found my way alone back to Paris and its most famous Jewish deli. Next to me four women my own age leaned toward one another, closing the space between them as they laughed and gossiped. So long as they were warmly close by I remained at my place and I kept ordering: chicken soup and matzo balls, a corned beef sandwich on rye bread, a plateful of sticky rugelach that I ate slowly, hungrily watching the women near me. I listened to them as they talked about going to the movies with their boyfriends and they laughed about the pressure that their mothers put on them to get married. "Goodbye!" they cried on the street to one another when they parted, and they hugged for many minutes under their wet umbrellas.

## 3

I try to phone my mother every day from New York. She's alone too much, and on many days the Chicago weather is too cold for her to venture outside. She still considers the cross-country call a special occasion: *long distance.*

If she's by herself, my mother may not bother with the hearing aids that never deliver the world to her quite as she knows it. I understand this, but when she asks me for the third time to repeat what I've just said, I bring my mouth close to the receiver and pronounce each word with hurting precision. When my mother asks if I think my sister is going to get another dog, I tell her roughly to ask Anita herself. And when she starts in on how she can't understand how corrupt politicians can live with themselves, I demand to know how she could be so naive. "That's what it's all about, don't you get it? That's the point of politics: *selfishness!*"

The next night it's my mother who calls back. She cuts me off before I can finish my first word. "Don't make me feel bad about myself," she says firmly into the telephone. "I'm not asking you that, I'm telling you."

"Goodbye," she says then, quietly, and we both hang up.

**4**

"Goodbye, Uncle Arnold," I hugged my uncle, ninety-one years old now, on my cousins' front sidewalk this spring. A soft wind was blowing across the snow-stripped stubble of lawn—the long midwestern winter finally giving way. "See you," he said to me, and he let go abruptly and headed back toward the house.

In the basement of their suburban Chicago bungalow, he and his three young sons spent long, patient weekends, forty years ago, working on the train set that ran along their ping-pong table. It was a wondrous thing to me: the tracks spilling over hills that my cousins plastered and painted, past the bristly evergreens they glued in clumps at sidings along the way; the striped warning gates that rose and fell on their own supply of electric power. As I descended the rickety stairs from the kitchen after my aunt had made us lunch, I could hear wheels making turns, metal against metal, and the train whistle sounding below, and I could feel myself approaching a boundary into the lucky world that my cousins and their father continually made and remade together. I loved how my uncle's workshop and office—the rows of tools hanging from pegboard and the massive gray metal desk stacked with files and folders—vanished from my line of vision as we hunched together over the trains, adding a bridge, waiting to see if each car would make the twists and turns on the figure-eight track without derailing. Smiling plastic families waved at the faces painted in the windows whipping by, and sometimes my own hand would rise to join theirs as the rushing air pushed me back from the edge of the table.

## 5

I silently enter my mother's garden before she wakes and we return to her closets. Alone here for the first time, I am astonished by what she's brought to life in this place and by what she will be leaving behind, still profuse and growing. Along the stone walk, rows of begonias—elegant, linen blossoms—are at their peak, set against the muscular darkness of waxy ground cover. In a large square at the center of the garden, a bold white border of impatiens surrounds delicate green ferns, and shiny leaves of hosta circle a high pot spilling blue bachelor's buttons.

Where was I when my mother was calculating for all this, when she was setting down the three ceramic frogs, half hidden in the thick of leaves during the blooming months, each one the size of her two clasped hands? Their eyes bulge over gaping mouths; next to them, a pair of ceramic birds sing on a piece of driftwood. A sheet metal crow—a single silver stake driven straight into dirt—spreads its gawky wings and stares out from brass nuts soldered to each side of its beak.

An invisible hand suddenly surprises my heart here, reaching for blood, pressing on muscle. Summer is ending, and the handyman has already stacked my mother's set of four chairs and turned her patio table on its side against the coming change of weather. This will be my mother's last garden, I think, where the seedlings she's started in clay and plastic pots will most likely wither while she is herself uprooted. My grandparents came to America from the small Jewish villages of Eastern Europe; from dark, gardenless places. In fifty years of seasons lived in this town, my mother has never bought a house without a garden, every one of them made hers by planting and tending.

"Don't open the curtains. I can't bear to see all the work that I'll never finish," she answers when I offer later, at breakfast, to pull the cord on the drapes that open onto the garden. My mother waves brusquely in the direction of the curtained window, and then turns away.

## 6

"Okay, kiddo," my mother says, as always, stepping back just a bit to take a last look at me before I pull out the handle of my rolling suitcase and head for the front door and the taxi waiting to take me to the airport, "call me when you get home." I take a long look at her too, wondering what exactly things will be like here when I next return.

It won't be long before the monarch butterflies start their migration, riding the earth's thermals. In one extraordinary trip, millions make it every autumn from Canada to the same twenty-mile square of Mexican fir trees, where they are so many that they pack the trunks and weigh down the hanging branches. And then the way back, three generations long; each generation a four-stage cycle from egg to caterpillar, from cocoon to adult. We used to watch the monarchs from our backyard when I was young, used to know the approach of winter from the soundless flocks that passed each year going south. A few always dipped close to us, and my sister and I would hold out our upturned palms, hoping to be touched by their magic, while my mother warned us to be gentle with the fluttering wings. "Goodbye," we'd wave from the porch as the last of the butterflies returned to the sky, and the air above us was emptied as quickly as it had been filled.

# In the Year of Masking Tape

My mother was born in the Year of the Ox. According to her Chinese horoscope, Oxen people are "often easy-going and trusting. But, on the other hand, they can also be stubborn, methodical." My mother has just sold the condo where she's lived for more than twenty years, across the street from the municipal health department where she ran the lab, a short drive from the synagogue where I went to Hebrew school and my sister and brother-in-law were married and my nephews and my niece had their bar and bat mitzvahs.

My mother and my sister and I visit our uncle Allan, dying two months into his diagnosis of pancreatic cancer. On a long table, jars of wrapped candy and nuts and dried fruit have been opened next to a stack of paper plates and a serving dish of stale jelly rolls: sorrow's anxious nibbling. A hospital bed has been set up next to the long picture window that too brightly lights my aunt and uncle's back room. We can see birds crowding the feeder outside that my aunt still keeps filled every day. Fat squirrels are chasing sparrows across the winter's fresh first snow in the yard, where my sister and I used to play with my cousins on the swing set and the jungle gym. On summer afternoons we'd fill my cousins' little pool from the hose at the side of the house and stretch out inside it, let the sun soak heat into our upturned faces. We'd listen to the squeak that the plastic walls of the pool made each time one of us got in or out, and try to coax my cousins' collie into the water with us. Or the dog would rest her long, heavy head on the swollen pillow of tubing until the wall collapsed and water spilled onto the grass and made mud in which we lay, happily, with her. When my cousin Gail was planning her wedding, she unfolded a map of Europe across this table and traced her honeymoon trip on it with her fingertips. My uncle and I clinked shot glasses and drank in her honor the burning Hungarian brandy that he loved. Now my uncle struggles to sit up, his beard bone white, his sweatshirt and sweatpants hanging from his shrunken body, and calls out softly to his attendant for help.

They are both Oxen, my mother and my uncle, both born— like Tony Curtis and Angela Lansbury—in 1925, the year that F. Scott Fitzgerald published his longing-loaded *The Great Gatsby*. In 1925 New York took over from London as the largest city in the world, Calvin Coolidge was inaugurated without a hint of the economic disaster ahead, John Scopes was tried in Tennessee for telling Charles Darwin's truth about the origin of human beings. More than sixty years ago, my mother and Allan were a couple, engaged to be married. As the Allies set final fire to Germany, my mother posed on her parents' front steps between two young men in thick eyeglasses, both too near-sighted to serve in the war, both ready to marry her—and then chose my father. While Gail and I hug and we cry together, my mother puts on her coat and zips it, raises the down hood against this bitter winter day. In her birth year, Benito Mussolini claimed absolute power over Italy and the painter John Singer Sargent died, ending a lifetime's work: watercolors of already fragile Venice and portraits of America's fresh successes. My mother turns toward the door, ready to move on.

My mother was born in the Year of Masking Tape, the 3M engineer Dick Drew's 1925 invention. At my mother's condo, pieces of the tan tape are wrapped like bandages around her travel alarm clock and around the radio on her bed stand. Tape crosses the clock's chipped housing where a missing tab has left a hole; I can feel the batteries bulging against my hand. The world broken and, at least temporarily, the world bound up. My mother's cell phone and her telephone handsets and the calculator on which she tracks her monthly budget are all striped with raw, lightly colored bits—so, she tells me, the dark plastic instruments will show up against her black countertops. The manufacturer rates masking tape by the number of days it can be left on without leaving a residue. Easy to tear, easy to remove, it was designed to do its work without leaving a scar.

In a few weeks my beautiful cat Sophie will be dying in a darkened room at the vet, trailing an intravenous drip. Warm as life in my arms, her taped furry leg tucked beneath her chest, her heart pressed against mine. My mother never liked Sophie, or her shedding on the furniture and on our clothes. "Here," my mother would demonstrate, forming a loop of masking tape adhesive-side out and rubbing the shoulder of my sweater with it. I'd follow the path of my mother's fingers across the fabric with my own hand, feeling for silky, beloved remnants of what she had swept away. When my father left her, my mother struggled to hold things together in the too-big suburban house that they'd bought together—built in the 1920s, when they both were born, miles from her family and the neighborhood where she'd grown up on the far side of the city. My mother packed up the house, and she unpacked and laid out our things in stacks in the first apartment that she'd rented on her own. Everything seemed smaller there, but my sister and I both held back for once from saying anything. Wounds we recognized that it was better not to reopen, softness over which we understood it was best not to linger, sadness it was better not to unseal.

Now, at my mother's new place, my sister and I slice through slick packing tape, its grip on the boxes too strong to be peeled free. Each box's cardboard surface is layered with names and destinations marked out in thick black ink, recycled from other people's journeys. We slowly unwrap the newspaper mummies that my mother taped shut in her old kitchen, the three-inch pair of rubber boots from Kew Gardens, London, and the clay pickle jar from Provence. I silently count one hundred thirty-three pens and pencils, sixty-seven of them brand-new in rubber-banded cellophane packages. Five spatulas. We try to convince my mother to give up the wingless Mexican painted birds, and the chipped owl. "That owl was Lucy's," she tells me, tightening her grip on her old friend's little statue. "Lucy collected owls, and when she died her kids gave them away. And—don't you remember?—we bought those birds on our trip to Oaxaca. I like to use them in flowerpots." My mother backs up against the dresser and holds her position.

My sister and I can be stubborn too, immovable as oxen, insistent when she moves here that our mother give up her car. From time to time, she pans anxiously from one side of the unfamiliar rooms to the other, trying to take stock of her losses, not yet fully taking in how her mobility has been wounded. She pulls out from one of the boxes a shellacked red Chanukah dreidel trailing a dirty cord and wooden cup. She fits the dreidel into the cup and sets the cup on her dresser. She turns to us and gestures decisively with one hand, stopping us from speaking: "Eddie and Ethan play with that," she says, and my nephew and my brother-in-law nod.

In the sixty-year Chinese astrology cycle, my mother's element is Wood, her color green, her season spring—the living world in metamorphosis. I can hear the wind picking up whistling speed in the street outside her apartment, the cars slowing down, some of them skidding in the quieting, accumulating snow. High in the heavens tonight my mother's zodiac planet, Jupiter, will emerge as always out of the dark, barely visible to humans in the distant, reflected light of the sun. And we go on unbinding boxes in the steamy, insular heat of what we all know will be my mother's last apartment, plugging in and turning on unpacked lamps as the windows darken and frost over. The purifying morning bath, the stripping down and letting go, the steering freshly clear: these were the rituals of Henry David Thoreau's hopefulness at Walden Pond, each day's radical accounting. Yet surely love's lingering, sweet residue is also right to cherish. Here, where the many, unnumbered years of life's wearing down are bound up with one another, all this is what is left to be reckoned with.

*Across the Serengeti, animals turn each year toward water, straining every muscle across miles of quickly drying grass, trailing a blowing swath of dust. At every point along the way, the flanks of the moving herds—the young who stray from their watching mothers; the old who stumble slowly along alone—are brutally picked off. The elegant beauty of the zebra is matched and ravaged by the cheetah; even the enormous elephant bears a look of panic when it takes in the fleet approach of death. Out from night's velvet blackness, the growling of lions reaches the wildebeests gathered shoulder to shoulder at a precious watering hole, telling them: nowhere is safe.*

# Mirror Writing

In April my mother told me that what was making me sad was my own mortality—and by July it turned out that she was right. I was rounding the corner on my fifth year of writing about my mother's chronic respiratory illness—and in a moment, without warning, I was facing the true fact that I could die before she did.

My plan had been to follow my mother's illness in the present tense, so that I could draw closer to her while she was actually living "end of life." I was hoping that by not waiting for the retrospective point when I could look back and read in reverse, I would create the potential for illumination. And indeed the limitations of my own freshly sixtyish anxieties about aging have been revealed to me by the way my mother has lived these years. For she has remained determined to wring whatever pleasure she can from each day rather than to peer ahead at death—a death that we all know could well take a painful, suffocating form.

My mother has proved to be stubborn, sometimes hilariously so (when she had to move out of her apartment, she refused to relinquish her stockpile of plastic margarine containers and her collection of mock turtlenecks—including the stained ones that she pulled out of the donation pile, announcing that she would just wear those backward). Yet she has also proved to be miraculously adaptable. She has faced, and accepted, 24/7 oxygen supplements, enduring the breathing cannula that hangs and hisses and makes her nose drip wherever she goes. She continues to play ping-pong with a five-pound oxygen tank slung across her chest.

So I had been learning from this writing project, and even acquiring an unanticipated humility: the effect of standing in attentive proximity to the unadorned courage required to live, and to breathe, every long day.

And then suddenly, late one summer afternoon, words began to drift out of my mouth on a trajectory of their own. It seemed at first like a stroke, though I was still *me* enough to weep at the thought of being carried on a stretcher at rush hour into an elevator crowded with my neighbors. Over the next days, I would become unrecognizable to myself: a person diagnosed with a potentially fatal blood disorder; forever a person with a scar on my neck—*"Insert here!"*—where the flesh was cut and a tube for total plasma exchange jammed into my jugular vein. If I was now someone whose life had been saved, I was also now a patient—as chronically ill as my mother.

How could I continue writing about my mother as though I were observing her from outside the circle of illness? During the last minutes before my neck was opened at the hospital, I waited on a gurney for a spent-looking woman to decide whether or not to continue medical measures to save her brother. She leaned against the wall and wiped her brow, opened her handbag and closed it, then turned to speak to one of the waiting doctors. Her visibly younger brother was wheeled out in silence as I watched, a stranger brought excruciatingly near to others' most deep pain. And then it would be my turn to be ushered into the circle.

It has been six years now since my diagnosis—six years since my mother and I strangely crossed paths with one another on what had seemed, safely until then, like two separate journeys. At the Passover seder this spring, my mother named "lack of forgiveness" as one of the Ten Plagues of our time. I love the capaciousness of that critique, how it speaks to my mother's lifelong determination not to bear a grudge, and the habit of acceptance that has without a doubt carried her through illness and its diminishments. But I am, myself, not yet ready to be so openhearted.

Recently I was invited to recite at my synagogue the traditional prayer of thanks for deliverance, the *birkat ha'gomel.* My instinct to keep starting fresh in my writing about my mother has led me, as I had hoped, to the heart of things: to the daily present in which my mother continues to love life. But for me the present remains tinged with uncertainty. In my household, *now* has come to mean *Since I got sick*. Over two summers I returned to the hospital in an ambulance four times; once after an adverse drug reaction during which I could not remember the day of the week or the season or the fact that I had just fed the cats—or even that I *have* cats. So I cannot yet claim to have put danger behind me. I cannot accept an invitation to closure.

Six months after my diagnosis, I returned with my wife to Sanibel Island on the Gulf Coast of Florida, where we had spent a week on a family vacation ten years before. On that earlier trip, we had shared a humid cabin on the shore with my mother, and laughed at the doggedness with which she trolled the beach every single day for the shells that Sanibel is famous for. Every inch of our bathroom and kitchen counters was covered by early morning with more shells than we could possibly take home, drying on paper towels: tiny conches, perfect and complete; pairs of butterfly shells, still delicately joined. On a shelf at home, we keep a big jar in which the shells that my mother and Ellen and I collected remain forever confounded with one another. We could not have guessed that a decade later it would be impossible for my mother to breathe on her own in the hot sun, or to bend to the sand for what the tide had left there—much less how the tides of my own blood would be disrupted.

As I unpacked the car trunk on our return trip to Sanibel, a white egret headed gawkily across the hotel parking lot—its long twin legs like knitting needles—then opened its big white wings and flew, took sudden, perfect flight like an angel over the dusty cars and the hot, sticky macadam. Following in my mother's wake with words keeps bringing me back as well to the ways in which the world goes on being stubbornly beautiful. And yet I can no longer pretend that the ragged approach of death is likely to be smoothed by nature's grace, or by the natural order. So long as I believed I was writing about my mother, I was able to hold mortality at a distance, to hold it—falsely—at bay. Now in the mirror of my mother's aging face I see myself.

# Written in Blood

"We are in uncharted territory now," my doctor cautions in the examining room, where I'm waiting as usual on a papered table, anxiously swinging my legs. He means that because my blood disorder is so rare, our only choice is to experiment with protocols developed for other illnesses: powerful, dripping therapies aimed at the immune system. I close my eyes for a moment and imagine myself as an astronaut. My bubbled head pans the landscape of an alien planet, my vehicle setting off clouds of dust as it lands and then takes flight again, returning to Earth with a discovery that will make medical headlines.

Or perhaps I've simply lost my way, like Álvar Núñez Cabeza de Vaca, whose Spanish crew was stranded on the coast of Florida in 1528, leaving him to walk for nine years along the Gulf Coast and into the interior of the continent. When their clothing wore out in the harsh sun and wind and the daily usage of years, Cabeza de Vaca and his handful of comrades went naked during the day and slept at night under deerskins. The indigenous people among whom they sought shelter came close to feel the Spaniards' unfamiliar faces and bodies, passing curious hands over the pale, sunburned European flesh. I roll up my sleeves and lift each arm so that my doctor can check for fresh bruising, a sign that my clotting system has once again gone haywire. I am wearing clothes but I feel exposed. I have become an object of curiosity, a mystery to be solved. I have fallen off the map.


For my sixtieth birthday, I got a rare autoimmune blood disorder—the kind that attacks unpredictably and without explanation until you die, unless you are lucky enough to have doctors who recognize the strange, seemingly unrelated symptoms that strike only a handful of people in a million. Thrombotic thrombocytopenic purpura (TTP) was actually named at the hospital where I arrived at the emergency room unable to put a sentence together—looking like I was having a stroke. In the ER, time comes untethered during the hours of procedures and tests and of waiting for results, surrounded by others' unceasing cries. The normal human blood platelet count is 150,000–400,000, and my count that "night" was 33,000.

Like other autoimmune disorders, TTP turns the body eerily against itself. Instead of defending against infection, an antibody attacks the enzyme whose job is to break down a protein in the blood. The large, sticky protein molecules that continue to circulate intact attract platelets and form clumps, dangerously lowering the count of circulating platelets essential to clotting, blocking vessels that provide blood to the brain and the kidneys, and causing anemia by fragmenting red blood cells.

Few outward signs reveal this betrayal of the body's own defense system until it has made bewildering headway. In my own case, I experienced a string of what my neurologist calls "visual disturbances." Without warning, a crescent sliver— finely layered like a fragment of mica—would appear before each of my eyes and slowly grow, blooming into the full spectrum of colors and drifting downward over my field of vision. The afternoon when speech suddenly eluded me, words and sentences defied my control like unleashed animals. After I had recovered my ability to talk, when the mysteriously blocked blood vessels to my brain cleared in the emergency room, a hematologist found the telltale bruising in the hanging low spots just above my elbows, where unclotted blood was collecting and pooling below the skin's surface.

Just twenty years ago, more than 90 percent of the patients diagnosed with TTP could expect to die; with treatment, more than 80 percent can now expect to survive. Total plasma exchange can save a patient whose blood would otherwise fatally malfunction. Plasma *pheresis* removes the patient's entire blood supply, centrifuging off the clearish plasma with its rogue antibodies and replacing it with fresh frozen plasma from healthy donors. During my hospital stays, I have been "pheresed" close to twenty times, my own plasma exchanged for—and exposed to—the plasma of nearly two hundred donors.

Forever now I will be wheeled, when my blood rebels like this, into the intensive care port lab, a glowing cube at the center of a constellation of curtained beds, beeping instruments, and hovering relatives. Each time, a gowned and masked figure will turn me on my side for a sonogram of my neck, measuring and mapping the way into my jugular vein. Cold anesthetic will be sprayed on my skin to prepare for the incision, a guide wire inserted to feel for the route to my heart. I will feel the dull *thunk* of plastic tubing follow, hitting its mark inside, and wait through the minutes during which stitching fixes into the flesh of my neck a double-ported catheter. Finally, before I can be pronounced ready for treatment, I will be rolled back through the hospital's shadowy basement corridors for an X-ray to confirm that the catheter that's designed to draw out and then replace my blood has been correctly placed.

As at so many other sites of intimacy between life and death, there is ritual here. In the hospital I wait every day for the pheresis nurse to appear with crumpled paper bags in each hand, to set the bags on the night table at my bedside and haul in the lumbering machine that must be positioned in the narrow space between my bed and the wall. When the floor nurse arrives, she reaches into the paper bags for plastic sacks of donor plasma, and the two nurses begin their chorus. For each bag, one voice calls out my name and my date of birth, and then each donor's blood type and a serial number. The other voice confirms, *Yes.* One by one, each thawing sack is hung with a metal hook from a bar on the big machine. The sacks dangle in a lengthening row. The pheresis nurse flips a switch, and the machine with its lighted dials makes an oddly primitive grinding noise. The nurse opens the catheter in my neck, uncorking me like a bottle.

For the next three hours, I will be at the mercy of another human being as I am emptied and refilled. I search through the television channels, hoping that a documentary on desert rock formations or the annual migration of sandhill cranes will divert my attention from the long tubes flowing red next to me, loaded with my lifeblood. Beside me the machine grinds and shudders, festooned with its web of tubing—spinning off the dangerous mistakes that my own body keeps making; warming the alien blood that we hope will become mine, that we hope will repair me.

"Are you in pain?" a nurse asks on my first morning in the hospital. "Pain changes everything." I am glad to be able to answer no, not only because I am relieved to not be suffering but also because I am not ready to see myself in the hurting bodies of the patients all around me. "Soon they won't even be able to control the pain," my roommate worries to me. A pleated curtain is hung between us, stirring whenever someone passes—marking the boundary between the two sides of the room as though it were only space. As my roommate hits the call button to request more meds, I slide to the far side of my bed, distancing myself from her unpitying, unstoppable pain.

I try to disappear into silence when doctors and nurses examine my roommate. I am angered by our closeness, reluctant to take off my clothes and risk rubbing naked against the bathroom walls that her skin may have touched, afraid to let my loose gown come in contact with the sink. I pull down paper towels and lay them carefully over the toilet seat before I sit down. I mimic the hospital staff, squirting my hands whenever I pass a Purell dispenser mounted to the wall.

Day and night I can't help overhearing from the other side of the curtain doctors telling other human beings that their lives will never be the same. "That's a hard load that you've given me," another roommate tells her brisk young doctor in her lilting African accent. "I am not sure I know how to bear it." Would turning up the volume on my TV be disrespectful—or just the right signal to transmit over the airspace between us my recognition that listening to this conversation is wrong? She begs the doctor to let her stay longer and face here among professional caregivers the pain that she knows—from many times before—is coming. When he leaves I tiptoe to the bathroom, and I can see that she has turned her face to the wall. Every day that we have shared this room, her best friend from their childhood in Senegal has come to her here, gently helping her to bathe and then to put on a fresh hospital gown—and taken the time to exchange a few words with me, to enjoy the friendly pretense that we are practicing my French together. When I wake in the morning, I find on my bed stand a gift from my roommate, two foil packets: a goo that breaks down the cloying adhesive residue left on every long-term hospital patient by tape and tubes and procedures. When she moans at night, though, I do not respond, I do not seek help, I do not try to ease her pain. We do not come here prepared to know one another.

Still, so many others approach me. In the lounge at the end of the corridor, a mother whose teenage son's cancer has returned after four years of remission stands for long minutes at the window looking out in the distance at the Hudson River, at the shimmering metal drawbridge crossing over water from this island of pain. When she turns, she touches my gowned arm and says that she hopes that things go well for me. A woman hangs back from her husband as he leaves the floor lounge to tell me that this is the fourth day in a row on which this limping elderly man has fasted since midnight before a surgery that has, once again, been canceled. "I thought I was going to lose her," another man, about my own age, turns to say to me, clasping and unclasping his hands. I had heard his wife crying in the dark, their three sons gathering one by one at her bedside and murmuring to one another.

"Good morning, Miss Joanne," the mother of yet another roommate, a young woman whose excruciating sickle cell anemia has relapsed, greets me. Scratching my dirty hair—outrageously bound in a bright pink band to secure the heavy pheresis tubing to my head—I am disbelieving when I catch sight of myself in the mirror. *If Pebbles Were Hospitalized*, I mentally title this image. "I think that you look beautiful," my roommate's mother says to me, standing back to take in the full effect and smiling. Each morning I review my body with fresh surprise. My arms are striped with colorful symbolic bangles and badges. On the right, first a wide blue band marked not only with my name but also the name of my doctor, not only my date of birth but also the date of my hospital admission. A clunky GPS device on the band reminds me that I am being tracked. Moving up my arm toward my elbow, a red bracelet is stamped with a warning about my food allergies, then a pink one, *Fall Precautions*. On my left hand, wrapped in thick clear plastic, an IV connection has already been threaded into one of my veins, ready to be deployed in an emergency.

Who am I now? Someone who is ill, someone who uses a bedpan. I try to control my intake of liquids so that I can avoid having to urinate during the long hours of plasma exchange.

For the first four treatments, I succeed—and then I give in and humiliate myself. One more way in which I have agreed to let my body be opened up to strangers.

My roommate's curious father pulls back the corner of the curtain between us to watch my treatment, staring at the rumbling machine that is siphoning off my blood. "This is not for the public," a protective nurse frowns at him, and he withdraws. One night an aide wakes me at 3 a.m. and packs up my small stash of belongings while I wrap my arms around myself in the hospital never-nightness, determined not to cry. They are moving me to the oncology ward, where the staff is better equipped to deal with my rare condition. I pad through the halls, wrapped in a pair of flimsy, wrinkled gowns back to front, incompletely sealed, exchanging stories about the hospital food with other patients in the lounge. I am one of them now. I wear the same uniform as they do.

To have been diagnosed with a chronic illness is to have become a stranger to myself. I am a writer of personal narrative whose body—receiving the confounding signals sent by autoimmune disease—no longer knows the difference between itself and its enemies.

Sometimes when I lie cocooned in my hospital bed with the curtains pulled tight around me, I can feel the force of my blood as it finds its path into every part of my body, taking disease wherever it goes—against my will—shearing red cells into fragments.

Blood, I am learning, keeps its own dictionary, a lexicon for what goes as deep as life, for what can hurt the most, for what is true about ourselves even if we don't yet recognize it. My blood is pulling me back into language, demanding revision.

*Blood sport*: a competition or a conflict whose stakes are as high as the maiming and killing of living things, as in hunting, bullfighting, and cockfighting.

*Blood pact*: an agreement between two individuals whose uniquely binding status is marked by the placement of blood from each party next to her or his signature. *Written in blood*.

To become chronically ill is to be pushed over a cliff—to be set into freefall. Waiting, the first time, on a gurney in the hospital basement, just barely understanding that my neck still needs to be X-rayed, the correct placement of the catheter stitched into my jugular vein not yet confirmed, I am nowhere, a patient without a bed, a displaced person. I do not grasp what lies ahead: the unstoppering of the tube, still a raw wound in my flesh, the release of my wild blood. Or the seriousness of this procedure: without it, I will die.

Above me a face appears, smiling and speaking, and I slowly realize that I know this man. This is the hematologist whose office I visited after my low platelet count was first discovered in the hospital emergency room. His name doesn't come to me and he can see that, so he tells me and I remember. He is explaining what will happen next, after the X-ray, and I only half listen, resisting as I will continue to do in the days ahead in the hospital and then the weeks and months at home, unready even to admit the full name for my illness into my vocabulary: *thrombotic thrombocytopenic purpura*. But I do grasp, as I sit up and face him in the shadowy corridor, that this man is now essential to what my life will be from this day forward, that he is part of my new life. The next morning, when he comes to visit me during my treatment, he lays his hand gently over mine.

It was only a few treatments into the plasma exchange cycle when the catheter through which all my blood needed to pass became blocked by sticky clotting agent. "Sometimes it's just a matter of positioning," the pheresis nurse explained, and she began to shift me in the bed like a long, lumpy pillow until she managed to find an angle at which blood could flow in and out again through the tube jammed into my neck. As the nurse rocked my body, then bent it into a giant *S*, I shut my eyes tight, miserably turning away from what she must be seeing: the gown riding up over heavy thighs, dirty hair spilling over the clumped sheets—a flailing doll inflated to nightmare size. Once things got going again—"We're in business!" she announced with cheerful relief, standing back—I found that I still could not open my eyes. I could hear the machine humming again, could feel the blood pressure cuff once more tightening and releasing, but I was realizing for the first time that even this treatment was not a guarantee. *What will we do when nothing works?* I began to wonder. The steroids that I could feel beating inside me escalated my panic, my sense of dropping over an edge. I was abandoned on a strange, fluorescent-lit planet, uselessly watching life as I knew it recede into the cosmic distance. I did not want to recognize myself there—as this.

The nurse starting up my next pheresis treatment arrived after midnight and fumbled for long minutes with a knot of tubing that he needed to insert into the sticky catheter. I could feel fright penetrating me, as cold as the thawing plasma. On the far side of the familiar, waiting behind my closed eyes, I imagined my veins filling with blood-colored dread. But when the nurse muttered to himself, "All I can see is bubbles," I sat upright and waved him away. "Stop now," I told him. "It's the middle of the night, and I've never seen you before. Don't touch me." *Do not touch my blood.* And he withdrew at my command.

In freefall you have to let go of the expectation—what you thought was knowing—that you can count on landing. And yet you also come, in that limbo, into new knowledge.

What an irony is the word *autopsy*: from the Greek "seeing with one's own eyes." I will surely not be privy to any vision of myself that others are able to discover, if ever my body is laid out and opened up for death's public mapping. And yet if that knowledge, whatever it may be, is withheld for so long as I live, many other secrets have already been rendered visible to me. To live with chronic illness is to *un-know* one's body as private, to un-know the end of healing as *cure*; to un-know the story one has been telling as one's own, to let go one's grip on the old, untested clarities that used to guide daily life. But it is also to *know* for the first time that the human body is a fluid, changing thing, certain to be disrupted.

A lot can go wrong during plasma pheresis. An incorrectly placed catheter can puncture a lung; if it is left in for too long, the catheter can become infected. Exposure to donor plasma can cause an allergic reaction, even send a patient into potentially fatal anaphylactic shock. During pheresis, a patient's blood pressure can drop precipitously. I have been one of the lucky ones, and these dramas have not, thankfully, become my story. Despite a relapse after my initial year of remission, we are seeing the good results that many TTP patients can only hope for from plasma exchange, and from the outrageously expensive, big-guns immunotherapy drug Rituxan, which my hematologist added to my treatment plan: the disappearance of the antigen that sets off the destructive autoimmune cycle, and the rise to normal levels of the enzyme that sustains the proper balance of blood platelets.

Yet if treatment turns me away from danger, it also re-writes me into the narrative of illness that I will now forever be a part of. When I have Rituxan treatments in my hematol-ogist's office, I sit in a small room with other patients hooked up to mysterious infusions. Anonymously we fall asleep to-gether, our chins dropping to our chests, copies of the *New Yorker* slipping from our laps to the floor, feeling the effects of precautionary dosages of Benadryl. (Rituxan, for example, is brewed from the genes of mice and rats, significant allergens.)

Through the Benadryl haze I can hear my doctor—whom I have come to love, with whom I have shared a year and a half of fear and hope; of favorite, beloved books; of intimate details of my body—laughing with his nurse in an examining room across the hall. I do not know even the name of the man I am sitting next to, tethered like me to a bag of magic, potent chemicals. I do not know his illness. But I know that this is my place, here next to him; that he and I belong together now.

"To the last," Cabeza de Vaca wrote in the *Relación* that he completed upon his return to Spain, "I could not convince the Indians that we were of the same people as the Christian slavers." Between the lines lay Cabeza de Vaca's secret journal of survival: his abandonment of the story of colonial domination that he had expected to write, and his taboo acceptance of the Indians as partners. Christopher Columbus kept his own secrets as well, two separate journals recording two parallel worlds: one, the route he had planned, toward India's spices; the other, a route to the islands of the Caribbean, not yet imagined on a map. In whom could Columbus confide? To whom could he reveal his fatigued uncertainty? I recognize the terror Columbus must have felt as he came unmoored in the universe, for his crew had put their trust in his navigational skills, counting on him against terrible odds to keep them safe, as stubbornly as the king and queen of Spain waited for investment in his journeys to turn a profit. In his third letter, Columbus finally let loose from the known map, fantasizing below the equator the glowing, uncrossable frontier of "the earthly Paradise"; laying out his own vision of a globe topped by a stalk "like a woman's nipple on a round ball." Columbus survived, but he returned to the court of Spain in humiliating chains. And still he refused to relinquish his story of having discovered a route to Asia.

On the hot, packed subway I clutch the railing, reading and rereading the bodies veering toward me at every shuddering stop, wary of invisible viruses, on the alert for contagious breath coming close. I no longer leave home unprepared, without my cell phone and my health insurance card. And the emergency medical identification card that I have fashioned, with a tiny red medical serpent printed out from a website—sending out its universal distress signal with my blood type, the name of my disorder, and my hematologist's contact information. I measured and cut the paper to fit into my wallet, scotch-taped it between pieces of clear plastic. From the Central Park Reservoir, where I pause on the walking path and spot my first soaring red-tailed hawk, I can also see the hospital on Fifth Avenue where I spent nearly a month over two successive summers.

On the map in my head, the borders of countries where they may not offer plasma pheresis treatments or where I would not trust the blood supply are now highlighted. I would be afraid to travel to the highlands of Vietnam, where I have seen in photographs the morning mist rising seductively over hidden lakes; or to return to Mexico, where I noticed for the first, hungering time just as I was leaving Oaxaca the quiet, shadowed archways brooding at the edges of churches and public squares. I have long hoped to visit Chaco Canyon, hulking and silent below the high desert sky; imagined the winding dirt road kicking up gravel on the long, slow way into the deserted ruins left in the echoing canyon walls by the Anasazi Indians. But one could not easily on that road reverse direction to find medical help, could not without skidding turn one's back on the sun rising over the ancient town—hundreds of years away from life. I still imagine my return to the towns of the Loire Valley, where I lived nearly forty years ago: to the ruined castle of Chinon, where a flapping peacock dropped with a harsh cry to the ground from a branch just over my head; to the medieval Abbey of Fontevraud, where among the shadowed tombs of Plantagenet royalty Richard the Lion Heart lies buried. At least for now, though, I can no longer allow myself to be called by mystery.

So long as I live, chronic illness will keep calling me back out of time, out of *chronos*, out of narrative's forward motion. Next time—for almost certainly there will be a next time, though we possess no certainty about its hour—thrombotic thrombocytopenic purpura returns, we will call it a "recurrence," a looping back. When that happens, I will sit on the edge of another hospital bed and slowly strip. I will remove the street clothes that belong to a life—the life in which I dared to imagine myself "well"—that I must once again reluctantly relinquish. My shirt, my pants, and my bra. The shoes that I do not want scarred by contagion. There are drawers for my folded clothes, I already know, in the little dresser that can be wheeled along with me, if necessary, to another hospital room. On the other side of time I will pull out these clothes and put them back on. But now, as time again abandons me, I will pick up from the foot of the bed the familiar hospital gown, unfold it, pull it over my shoulders, reach around my back for the inadequate ties, and face this self in the mirror once more.

In the hospital there may be talk of numbers, and warnings against unrealistic expectations, but deep in the blood fantasy flows, uncharted: lonely, lonely; loyal to its own stubborn, secret story of survival. To be confronted with the body's fragility is surely a loss, but it is also a revelation—forcing to the visible surface, like lava at first too hot to touch, the truth that illness is not just a detour but rather a set of markers along the course on which all of us, breaking down, are bound. In one's medical file the images collect: the soft whites and grays of bones and organs set against darkness in X-rays; the layers of brain tissue disassembled and rearranged by magnetism in each set of MRIs. Each of us leaves our wake of clues for doctors to attempt to put together, like the blur accumulating around horses and runners in motion in Eadweard Muybridge's pioneering photographs. The numbers mount in stacks of test results: blood pressure and oxygen levels, red cell and platelet counts, at once fact and enigma. The scales fall away, and there you stand revealed, blood pumping to the most remote reaches of your body, struggling to find its way.

# Resignation

Where can we take my mother, still just as eager to see life as she was when she could walk miles up long sets of steps and down museum corridors where the planet's curiosities are preserved under subdued light; fragile, centuries-old mummies in glass cases and solemn, whiskered catfish barely stirring along the graveled floors of big tanks? The world still beckons, but now she must rely on others to take her to it: to drive to the handicapped entrance and drop her off; to park the car and then wait with her in line.

Inside Chicago's Shedd Aquarium are the sea's most strange creatures, delicate and fierce. Barely flesh at all, jellyfish can trail tentacles as long as one hundred feet, can coast the ocean's warm currents for miles, breathing symbiotically through algae if they enter deep zones where the oxygen supply is low; can sting and kill human beings. My mother is less than five feet tall, and she is carrying an oxygen tank that weighs five pounds. Arthritis has slowed her stiff body. *Take me*, my sister and I know she will say if we tell her about the jellies exhibit, but it is too much for us to face, more than we are willing to do. The screaming kids, the fish-shaped french fries ground underfoot; the hard work of salvaging excitement, and of seeing her so changed. It will always be our secret how we refused life's late offerings, how we said no without saying a word, how we turned away from our mother without letting her know why we felt we had to.

*When I look at water, I see what I used to be, before I breathed air. Blood as warm and salty as the sea in which I swam still runs inside me, the body's echo of history that I cannot remember. Particles that have left their traces in me and in the raw universe through which they blow; matter that will never be lost though no one can any longer name its source.*

# If My Disease Were an Animal

To be diagnosed with a rare disease is to have wildness pressed upon you. You are not exactly the shy quarry that birders travel the world to add to their checklist—more like something sighted with surprise, something that no one was looking for and no one is completely sure how to handle, taken into tentative, uncomprehending captivity. Other diseases are receptive to medicine's domestication. But yours rattles the bars of the hospital cage, breaks the rules, raises eyebrows.

My illness connects me to the wild places where medicine itself is still a feral thing—untamed as tropical sunlight and flooding water. In the Amazon rainforest, healing is still rooted in the mysteries of what grows and flowers, in the bark of the cinchona tree—the source of quinine used to combat malaria—and in the leaves from which shamans brew the psychedelic *ayahuasca*.

Now I too am possessed of visions. Fruit of the jungle yucca, corticosteroids drive away sleep, fill me with wild energy, exhaust me. Bells sounded by patients in pain too sharp to bear alone, or in trouble that they cannot understand, penetrate the half-dark, half-quiet night surrounding my hospital room. I dream of going home, I dream of being healed, I dream of my clothes rising out of the battered chest of drawers at the side of my bed where I exchanged them for a worn cotton gown—hardly enough fabric to cover my shame in daylight—and draping me, making me whole again. In my dreams my blood is still as good as the blood of the nurses who sample my veins and the doctors who track my platelet counts, the shamans who hold the power to keep me here. I imagine unhooking the tubes that connect me to machines, of leaving them opened and dripping—of fleeing through the long hospital corridors, down the elevator emptied of patients and visitors and flapping white coats, to the streets that will reabsorb me into the unceasing life of the city.

If I have met my match, I would like for it to be a thing of muscled beauty, reflecting back to me the grace and resilience possessed by only a small number of creatures. Fewer than seven thousand snow leopards survive in the remote highland forests of central Asia, still, as always, living to kill. Hunters pick them off one by one for their gorgeous spotted pelts, yet only a few human beings have witnessed a snow leopard in the wild. Nor will many doctors ever encounter a patient with my disease, for it strikes only five to seven people in a million. And no one knows when my disease will return from hiding, for when I am in remission even a microscope cannot find evidence of it in a smear of my blood.

Day approaches from the edge of darkness, one bed at a time floodlit as a soft voice announces, *Vitals*. What's "vital" has been distilled in the hospital to the small world of the body: down to temperature, blood pressure, oxygen ("blood ox"), pulse; a cuff placed silently around an arm, first squeezing and then releasing; a thermometer in an ear, a device clipped over a fingertip; a gloved hand feeling for faint pumping at the wrist, counting. Fitfully the signs of ordinary daily life return, the fidgeting wheels on linoleum, the steamy aroma of eggs and sausage uncovered on trays, the voices of the morning news rising from televisions with the sun.

The city is barely visible at dawn through my corner of hospital window. Alone in my bed, I imagine mist slowly burning away and leaving only trees and unmown grass. Out of the shadows, a lioness reaches her long legs and stretches, arching her roughly furred back, and looks at me, wrapped in a flannel sheet. She knows me, and she knows where to find me.

I am on a mission, flying alone into unfamiliar territory. I am a medical pilgrim, bearing the baggage of my rare condition.

In the airport at my destination, museum-size screens hang over the escalators, welcoming travelers who have come from far away to seek out specialized medical help. Beneath enormous block letters naming the clinic where I'm headed is a picture of a smiling, gowned patient, completely bald: visual shorthand for *cancer*. But this is not me; this is not my disease. At the curb outside, I watch an elderly couple board an airport shuttle to the Sleep-Eze motel. Some sort of device is dangling from her neck. *What's wrong with her?* I wonder. She looks tentative as she climbs the steps into the van one by one, taking long breaths as she goes, checking behind her for her husband. Has she come to this place, like me, hoping to stay alive? And is this how I look, at the airport information kiosk, at the front desk of my hotel: like a passenger coming, desperate, to the end of the medical line?

I follow a map of the giant medical school campus to the lecture room where I am to join a support group for others diagnosed with my disease. I find a spot at a table near the front of the room, sit down, and unpack my little notebook and my pen. Everyone in this room knows what I know, everyone here knows what it's like to live with the uncertainty of when, or where, or if, a relapse will occur. They know about the big machine that siphons off your blood, centrifuging it and replacing the tainted plasma with healthy plasma from donors. They know what it feels like to pass long days waiting for treatment, and then to wait for the results of blood work to reveal if your platelet numbers are rising from the scary lows that might already have caused organ damage. They have all wondered what their next hospital roommate will be like— friendly? moaning in pain through the night? accompanied by loud relatives who will ignore the sign saying that the bathroom in this room is for patients only?—and what the dinner they ordered will really turn out to be when they lift the silver dome on the tray. I wonder how many of them can, like me, call up in a second the remembered smell of disinfectant and the sound of mops in the hall at the end of the day, the stale sound of television seeping from every doorway along the corridor, almost an aroma clogging the air.

Off to the side of the lecture room is a table on which bottles of soda and bags of potato chips have been laid out alongside shrink-wrapped sugar cookies studded with colored jimmies. Folks all around me are forming a line that twists around the table, taking plastic cups and filling them, picking up napkins and loading their paper plates, while I watch, immobile—weighted down by disappointment. Could such pale, ordinary stuff be what's on offer today, on this occasion when patients with our rare diagnosis have journeyed from so many distant places? Can this be what we feed on when we gather, finally, together?

Day and night in cyberspace, families comb the universe for others like them who are suffering in isolation. They exchange symptoms—an infant son whose muscles are too flaccid to answer a hug; a toddler's mysterious failure to grasp a spoon; the itching that will not free them for even an hour—like playing cards whose matching suits must, they pray, be out there, somewhere. Hope depends for them on breaking out of the cocoon of solitude. The National Heart, Lung, and Blood Institute provides an online alphabet of "rare heart, lung, and blood diseases" on which it has compiled information: Klippel-Trenaunay-Weber syndrome (KTWS); supravalvular aortic stenosis (SVAS); lymphangioleiomyomatosis (LAM). On the website of my own disease, thrombotic thrombocytopenic purpura (TTP), I read: "We are stronger TOGETHER!" February 28, 2015, will be the next RARE DISEASE DAY USA, sponsored by the National Organization for Rare Disorders (NORD), its motto: "Join together for better care!" The director of the organization dedicated to my disease has driven through the night from Toronto to central Ohio to speak at our meeting and to hand out red rubber bracelets stamped *TTP* that each of us can wear to remind ourselves: *I am not alone.*

I stretch the bracelet hesitantly over my clenched hand, snap the band against the tender flesh on the inside of my wrist, against the blue veins through which blood is returning to my heart from my extremities. In the food line, others are shyly beginning to trade stories: comparing their first episodes, comparing their relapses, comparing treatments; sharing the sense of anxiety that never entirely abates, and the ongoing confusion of reading their own bodies. But I hold back, reluctant to see myself in their faces, unwilling to step away from the rare glow that is illuminating me, unready to be dis-enchanted.

If my disease were an animal, what would it be?

Would it be a bird of prey, an eagle dropping without warning from the sky, its talons—the surprising source of the great bird's power—gripping what's alive and taking it away? The word "raptor" derives from the Latin *rapere*: to seize by force. The harpy eagle is strong enough to carry off a monkey. In the night, the great horned owl slowly pivots its head 270 degrees, planning, seeing what cannot see back. The owl's hearing is so acute that it can register sounds of prey moving beneath the earth's surface, the scrabbling of fleeing field mice. The vulture's survival depends on the knowledge he logs from the air: the migration of quarry that other predators kill and leave in the high grass, opened and bloodied, when their appetite is sated; the places where light sharpens as autumn gives way to winter and the stripped trees reveal the most vulnerable life on the ground.

My disease finds me without warning, assailing me, throwing me on the defensive. No one knows its cause. In the emergency room, my clothes are taken from me, my blood drawn, the pumping of my heart measured from a flimsy cot, barely set off from others' raw, animal cries and threats fueled by pain and by fear. I will be wheeled through long, dull corridors into the blinding lights of surgery, where a masked stranger will carve my living flesh, open a path into my warm throat, locate the blood circulating deep below the surface.

We imagine the hospital as a vast cityscape where human beings masterfully wield science against illness—corralling it, mounting it, riding it to its demise. But rare diseases remain wild things, animals on the loose, never not dangerous, the essence of *disease* itself. Doctors wield instruments, dispense pills, miraculously push sickness back from the ledge where it has cornered mortally ill people. But my disease holds its ground, continues to flirt with danger.

Over the past two years I have been re-wilded, forced to accept the animal truths of my human body. I have witnessed my own blood drained, exposed to day's light, mixed with the plasma of strangers—turning me back to the elemental raw-ness that few must face, much less see, in themselves. I have been crazed by the careening high of prednisone—adrenaline untasked, the body's own steroid set loose so that it can mus-cle every moment to emergency-level power. Before my eyes my body has been disassembled, revealed as possessed by an alien force. My doctor presses the cold disk of his stethoscope over the thin fabric of my gown, listening for the brute, animal heart—just a beating thing, really, driven by surging blood and by the untamable urge to survive.

But if the diagnosis of a rare disease means consignment to wildness, it is also a call to the imagination. In my hospital bed, I devour books about ravens, birds of perfect blackness, of mysterious, glossy sheen, their dark eyes seeming to signal recognition. The condor—a carrion-eater like the raven—sails the updrafts of the Andes, alert for carcasses of large animals like deer and cattle. Yet even with its soaring ten-foot wingspan, the condor remains an ugly thing, with a vulture's featherless head. I envision my illness, instead, as a luminous raven: called like the vulture and the condor by fresh blood. Like their relatives the magpies and crows, ravens are smart and engaging, thieving employers of strategy. The Haida of the Pacific Northwest have elevated the raven to the mythic status of a trickster who teases human beings and challenges them, reflecting back to them their own nerve and creativity.

From the deck of a nineteenth-century whaling ship, humans could see the big beasts riding the water, their flesh scarred by encounters with predators, beating maimed fins, dangling embedded harpoons. On their bodies the relentless pitch of survival was made visible to the naked eye, and the dark threat of the unknown. Though he survived his fall overboard into the roiling sea, Herman Melville's deck boy Pip was forever altered in *Moby-Dick* by the sight of "God's foot upon the treadle of the loom."

Nor can I return to the certain, safe place I came from. Two decades ago I peered over the gritty rim of the universe at the Grand Canyon, into the void where what time and water can do even to solid rock is revealed. But I am no longer a tourist of boundaries. Illness is a wild dream, remote as the far edge of night from what we think we know. And when it envelops us, when it fogs and transforms ordinary life, we can only hope—I see now—to emerge a little more fully awake.

On summer days at our neighborhood Lake Michigan beach, my cousins and I used to tiptoe to the sand's edge, daring one another toward the lapping water. We'd enter in a wobbly line, shivering, our still incompletely formed bodies warmed from the waist up by the sun. And we'd pause in unison, aroused by what we knew would happen next. The sudden immersing cold—an electric, hurting chill—would take us in an instant past the string of floating buoys, to the faraway shores of the three-hundred-mile-long lake and the Canadian frontier that still glowed with Indian and French names. Petoskey (from the Ottawa *Pet-O-Sega*, or "Rays of the Rising Sun"), where beautiful bits of fossil coral continue to surface after millions of years. Mackinac, Sault Ste. Marie: places where ships loaded with beaver pelts docked, shaggy with ice after long travel from the north woods. Lucky, lucky us to be able to walk from our own backyards to the greatest of inland seas, chattering with one another as we floated toward the vast interior of the continent scooped out by massive, slow-driving glaciers.

To be diagnosed with a rare disease was never my intention—who among us would hope for such a destiny? I am marked for life as a medical curiosity. The treatments my doctor orders constitute the most sober of guesswork. Residents crowd my hospital bed for a look at a patient with my diagnosis. I stare at the blood that fills the tubing in the technician's gloved hand, subtly tinted in a secret code that even I don't know. Unlikely to profitably repay investment in research, rare diseases are easy, I have come to know firsthand, to abandon: medicine's "orphan diseases." Still, I do not mourn my fate as one of the stars in God's firmament that slipped out of alignment. "Rare," precious, unique, valuable, unlikely, unprecedented: Who would I be now, without this drama and this mystery?

My double-scarred neck reveals the fang marks of surgeons' scalpels seeking the jugular, seeking—to save me—the same route to the heart that any killing animal hopes to open. Southeast Asia's Hmong tribes honor the epileptic, shaken free of the ordinary, as a seer. I too have been seized by a great force, brought into the presence of pounding uncertainties. Twice already my disease has taken me to the brink, where the creaky workings of life are laid bare and forced into the light—at once sweet and bitter, unwelcome and amazing. Like a raven my disease takes flight, taking me—taking me with him. He scares me, he enthralls me, he grips tight my attention, he takes me on a wild ride to a place where I cannot count on surviving. I cry out, I growl, I claw my way back to life, strangely renewed. Wings dark as night, eyes bright as stars, my most intimate enemy and my most inscrutable companion, he comes back for me again and again.

# Dead Reckoning

*in memory of*
*S. V.*
*1952–2009*

From the plane slowing in the sky, Chicago's high-rises appear, clustered at the lake's edge: Oz shimmering in winter. And then the drive from the airport, past squat strip malls and blocks of split-levels, each blond facade plastered with a layer of lumpy stone. The snow that fell a day or two ago is already dirty in the street, piled up at the edges of gas stations and convenience store parking lots. I can remember when the McDonald's signs first flashed at these intersections the astonishing news: "One million sold!" At close range, time's tarnishing wake settles and clings.

I ring my mother's bell and she slowly comes to meet me. Behind her front door a machine pumps, distilling oxygen from air. My own lungs fall into the thrumming motor's pulse, filling and emptying; the unthinking alchemy of living. In my mother's apartment, it's the sound of death being pushed mechanically away that is audible to me now—steadily asserting its nearness, setting a known course.

My friend Sarah is my age and she is dying, at home in Vermont. "We had a bad night," her former partner Karen, come to care for her at the last, tells me when I call. Karen's voice drops so low that I have to guess at what she's saying, piecing together what I can catch and comprehend as though it were a foreign language: the intestinal blockage that nearly always brings ovarian cancer to a starving close; the thirst that ravages when the body can no longer absorb anything but an occasional handful of ice chips; the retching that fills the night even when the digestive system is completely empty. Outside, the cold is steadily emptying everything as well, stripping the trees and sucking the moisture out of the air. And still Sarah will not let go. "Maybe I should have agreed to one more round of chemo," she rasps in the night, leaving Karen in despair. Karen cannot convince Sarah to say yes to morphine's easing; to open her heart to death.

I can't find a working pen in my mother's kitchen, but she has her own system going on there. She stops me with her arm at the counter's edge, where I'm headed with my oatmeal bowl, and points: the soft stuff goes down the disposal, the plates and mugs get just a rinse on one side of the sink and then are stowed in the plastic dishrack on the other, until enough of them accumulate for a load in the dishwasher below. She pulls out a long drawer to show me the double layers of plastic bags, the little bags for the wet rubbish that she ferries daily out to the trash before it starts to rot and smell, the bigger one for the lighter loads that she can still manage a couple of times a week. Eggshells, coffee grounds, grated ginger exhausted in hot tea—all set carefully to dry on a dented aluminum pan to the left of the sink; mulch for her garden. Used paper towels drying on the rack, shopping bags in the corner filling with paper and bottles and cans. Her days cycle in succession, paced by pills and back exercises and breathing treatments and family visits.

At night my mother and I play Scrabble together on her kitchen table. I stare at the worn squares lined up along my wooden rack, impatiently arranging and rearranging them, but they won't make words. "You're too tense!" my mother tells me as the minutes pass after her last turn. "It's just a game!" Her letters clack in a triumphant line across the board, picking up points in every direction. I sit back in one of the kitchen chairs that my mother salvaged from the house in which I grew up, the chairs that have followed her through four moves, and I close my eyes. I feel the closeness of uncertainty—a cold jelly infiltrating my limbs—as though I've driven down a flooded road where the water's lapping boundary is marked only by a blank cone.

"I'm fine," my mother tells me when I phone from home in New York a week later. "I've got plenty to do today, more than enough to keep me busy." Today, when the cold is not so bad, she is going grocery shopping. She'll see what's on sale, what kind of fruit is cheap in the Chicago markets in the dead of winter, what brand of frozen green peas has been marked down at the A&P: the narrowing economy of going on. I imagine her lifting the heavy brown bags and unloading them on her kitchen counter. Then she'll have to lie down and rest, get her breath back. On TV I watch a gull turning slow circles over the ocean's edge, its patient wings making the wind do the work of waiting until it spots what it's hungry for. The gull drops headfirst to the sand and rises, a shuttered clam in its beak—dropping and retrieving and dropping again from high in the air until the heavy shell splinters on the rock below, leaving moist, helpless flesh exposed on the sunny beach. A male penguin loses his hold on the egg that he's cuddling and it rolls away, bumping and breaking on hard ice; instantly he reaches in the arctic wind for the egg that's tucked precariously into his neighbor's warm feathers. Loss is the currency of survival, I know, but witnessing is too much for me to bear.

When Inuit hunters have finished harvesting a bowhead whale carcass, they return the stripped skull to the sea, letting the whale's spirit go free. I can see how people with such beliefs can make themselves ready for death. "That's the road we travel," a man tells a young television interviewer after a member of the chorus in which he sings—men and women in their seventies and eighties and nineties—dies the night before the concert for which they've been preparing for months. My mother is traveling that road too, moving at her own pace, saying only what she needs to say. Her way is the way of doing until there's no more to be done, not the way—my way—of words.

It is nearly the shortest day of the year when I visit Karen in New Jersey after Sarah has died. Over the train heading back to Manhattan, the moon is hanging just shy of full in the sky, a hunk of rock suspended in black, barely lit by what's left of the afternoon's sun. Ahead, on the other side of the invisible Hudson River, the Empire State Building burns in the night, a green tube topped by glowing red. From here the human world—train tracks and bridges and buildings—seems implausibly laid out across the planetary crust.

On the plains lightning sets the high grasses ablaze in summer, and life burns before it can begin again: field mice trapped in their burrows, and fleeing deer; the densely seeded clover pods swaying in warm wind that my mother and I marveled at on a decades-ago visit to a tiny fenced prairie being called back from extinction along the lakeshore. It was still spring when my mother knelt in the sandy soil, bringing her face close to the pink shooting star blossoms that hung, nearly weightless, from the smooth stalks. She took deep breaths of their juicy fragrance while our guide explained that these flowers, unique to the prairies and to this season, would be gone by the end of June, when the plants would wilt in the hot sun down to their roots, thick and tangled as dry veins.

# My Mother, Gardening

"Can you see anything inside?" his companions cried out to the archaeologist Howard Carter when he opened King Tut's tomb, secreted in the sands for thirty centuries. "Yes!" Carter called back. "Wonderful things!" It was two and a half years before my mother was born. Carter and the others dizzily wandered the chambers where the young pharaoh had been buried, his sandals exquisitely carved; braided in solid gold to simulate woven reeds. All of Tut's organs, his heart and his liver, each kidney and his stomach, were embalmed and laid in stoppered canopic jars, then fitted into golden coffinettes. Coffers of fish and assorted meats; thirty jars of wine; four complete board games; one hundred thirty-nine ebony, ivory, silver and gold walking sticks; fifty linen garments—for the Egyptians believed that earthly human affairs continued in the afterlife—were preserved in the airless, crowded rooms.

I wonder what my mother would wish to take with her on such a journey, a journey beyond time. Surely she would hope to leave behind the damaged lungs that slowed her down in her eighties, though she has already lived so much longer than the Boy King, dead at nineteen. Without a doubt she would have her Scrabble board folded up and set beside her, the soft cotton sock still filled with worn tiles, the little wooden racks on which she'd sorted and re-sorted so many letters, made so many words. Her tennis racquet, just in case strength and flexibility should be granted to her once again. Perhaps she would keep the autumn leaves that I ironed in grade school between sheets of waxed paper and cut into bookmarks; and the clove-studded oranges that I made with my Girl Scout troop, as shrunken and fragrant as the aged, perfumed offerings surrounding Tut in his tomb.

And she'd want to take the flowers she had gloriously preserved all her life: the light blue salvia that she'd grown and hung to dry in pipe-cleanered bunches over the kitchen sink, the Queen Anne's Lace that she'd collected on weekend walks in the country. She always saved the loveliest of the roses from gift bouquets, at Mother's Day and birthdays, and gently sank them one by one into finely sifted sand. When she drew them out, the fragile blossoms would be perfectly fixed, hovering forever at the grayish edge of pink. *Wonderful things.*


In their first spring of suburban homeownership, my parents drove the six-lane Lake Shore Drive hugging Chicago to the annual flower show on the south side of the city. From the back seat of the car, my sister and I watched Lake Michigan's just-thawed water lapping crystalline along the entire route. On view at the vast McCormick Place were the newest innovations in home gardening: riding lawn mowers; racks of seed packets inviting amateurs to grow eggplant and other exotic vegetables; trowels, hoes, pruning shears; wheelbarrows scaled to suburban backyards and weekend work; peat containers that stretched the growing season by making it possible to start flowers and vegetables indoors. The end of wartime rubber rationing had already put giant coiled hoses into the hands of millions of optimistic home gardeners. My mother and my father entered a hungry trance as soon as they crossed the threshold of the exhibition hall and came into the presence of Burpee and Scott, the great merchandisers who'd plastered the long walls behind their booths with enormous photographs of gardens in bloom and of flawless green lawns flowing infinitely into the distance. These were the dreams with which my parents loaded our car and drove home along the lakeshore—that inspired them to plan and to plant.

The Yellow Climax marigold—capable of growing as tall as three feet, of producing giant blossoms as wide across as five inches, of blooming as long as twelve weeks—was the Burpee Seed Company's featured hybrid in 1958, the year that my mother planted her first garden at the house she and my father bought together. At the height of summer, my mother would clip the luxurious marigolds she had successfully grown from seed, handfuls of intense yellow bobbing in the hot wind, reaching above her waist. She'd dip them in wax so that they would outlast the season. The marigold was the personal passion of David Burpee, the son of the company's founder—who became a registered lobbyist in 1960 so that he could campaign in Congress to name the marigold the national flower of the United States. My mother bought seeds from the glossy catalogs Burpee pumped out during the years following World War II, showcasing a series of brand-new floral hybrids whose very names exuded drama and expectation: the Yellow Climax marigold, followed by the Double Supreme hybrid snapdragon in 1960, and the Firecracker Zenith hybrid zinnia in 1963. When Burpee's plants blossomed in my mother's garden— luxurious flesh in pink, yellow, orange, white, and red—they transformed the day.

Arthritis and chronic lung disease have now, half a century later, made it impossible for my mother to bend to the level of dirt and plants, and to breathe outside during Chicago's humid growing season. This year my mother has twice had to be hospitalized for a week or more when pneumonia clogged her lungs and could only be reached by intravenous antibiotics. Since she sold the big house that she owned with my father, and the townhouse and then the apartment that she bought on her own after their divorce, these have become the new obligations of her hands: filling her oxygen tank; opening the spigot and listening for the sound of gas sucked into the vacuum; turning back the handle until she can hear the seal clicking safely closed. Her palms hug the metal for an extra second or two; she brings her ear close to listen for escaping air before she sets the little tank in its sling. In the open air of a car or in my sister's kitchen, evaporation steadily empties even the spare oxygen tank that my mother takes everywhere, filling her with anxiety. She chops the air for emphasis as she speaks, as though her words too could disappear, could evaporate into the greedy air and leave her stranded.

Winter's cold, spring's wind, summer's heat keep my mother indoors. When I visit I sometimes find her slumped at night in the bathroom chair where she sits for her inhalation treatments, her little masked face sunk to her chest. "It's OK, I'm fine!" she reassures me when I prod her, panicking that this time she will not wake up. She carries a saucepan to the breakfast table and unselfconsciously eats her morning oatmeal directly from it, saving the few steps and the breath that searching for a bowl would cost her. Her spoon clanks against the old, dented metal of the stainless steel Revere Ware that she and my father received as a wedding gift.

It has been more than five years since my mother could care for her condo garden. But now she is delighted to be gardening once again, here where she has been assigned her own small plot, raised to waist level so that she won't have to stoop. When I walk out with her, my mother points proudly to what's hers, sweeping her hands, purpled from the many blood draws that have left too much stale leakage to be reabsorbed by her aging veins.

High stalks of pink snapdragons hang over the tiny garden, their buds at once lush and delicate, more of them waiting to open at the top. Nasturtiums and zinnias—and, as always, marigolds—flash orange and yellow, summer's richest colors not yet flattened by the harsh midwestern sun. She steers me around to see what her seventy- and eighty- and ninety-year-old neighbors have grown nearby: dense clusters of flowers, strategically selected to attract monarch butterflies; aromatic strings of blooming tomato plants. Across from my mother's plot is an elegant Japanese garden, rocks laid out beneath the gnarled branches of bonsai evergreens, a dark square of sand absorbing sunlight, the created universe in miniature.

I roll down the window on the taxi ride from my mother's place to the airport, letting my hair fly in the wind. This busy road is lined with flowers, Parks Department plantings and surviving fragments of what used to grow wild here. Milkweed bobs in the narrow rectangles of green at the curb, releasing fluffy pods that coast across the sidewalk and float, heedlessly, into traffic. A meadow bird—a finch?—suddenly flaps upward from the rough grass and takes off into the late summer air. It's still surprisingly easy to peel back the surface of things here, to see that these suburban streets and strip malls have been carved out of living prairie and fields.

In the years before air conditioning, when she first was single again, my mother would steer us out of the city to the thick aroma of freshly mown grass. Morning's early heat whipped between the cranked-open windows as we rode onto the highway, the ramp's arc slowly turning us, finally pointing straight ahead. What sweet distances we covered in those days, tunneling into the wind at eighty miles an hour, the rush all around us too loud to make talking worth the effort, the AM radio crackling as reception came in and out, goldenrod passing in a blur as we moved down the forever stretch of asphalt under the dome of heaven. Only the mileage postings broke our sweep across Illinois and Wisconsin, toward the Mississippi and toward the Minnesota border: *Rockford 55; Milwaukee 29; Minneapolis–St. Paul 275.* At lunchtime we would stop at a roadside table to eat the tuna sandwiches and celery sticks that my mother had packed, stretching our stiff legs over the rough wood of the sun-soaked benches. Velvet cattails swung back and forth in the low ditches nearby.

In Eden, it was God's voice—"Where are you?"—that called Adam and Eve back to their bodies. They were not just deep in the garden, they suddenly realized with alarm, but intimate with it, their own delicate, fresh skin close to the plants and trees growing there, brushing directly against rough stems and leaves. "I heard the sound of you in the garden," Adam tried, lamely, to explain, "and I was afraid, because I was naked." In that place, no longer untouched by time, their human flesh was revealed among the blossoming trees for what it really was: a fragile servant of appetite; mortal, likely to be wounded. The garden, as well, was revealed as vulnerable to violation, unequal to its own promise. And yet, many generations later, Eden would still color the prophet Amos's imagining of release from exile: "My people Israel . . . shall rebuild the ruined cities and inhabit them. . . . They shall make gardens and eat their fruit." What lonely men they must have remained! Wandering ministers of abandoned gardens, their fantasy of remaking the wounded world forever threaded with anger and doubt, layered over an unyielding assurance of abandonment.

Even today, when her movement must be frugal, her breath slowed, my mother seeks out her garden in the morning coolness. She carries a trowel, and plastic bags from the grocery store that she's saved to collect weeds and dead flowers. She pauses when she comes to the end of the path, assessing what has grown in the sun since the day before, and slowly circles her plantings. She disconnects the oxygen tubing when I ask to take a picture: that is not who she wants to be, especially here, where she has renewed in her last years her refusal of loss. She does not think about dying, she tells me when I ask, nor does she think ahead many mornings beyond this one. My mother has no interest in death's deals, in giving up even a little of the time remaining to her in order to set aside beloved objects for a chanced afterlife, much less to furnish a lavish tomb; in sacrificing even for a moment the gift of *now* that she has been granted.

She gently cups a low, fresh flower, something that wasn't open last time she worked in this modest garden. Isn't this what we all dream of, the promise of forever starting over, the human means of making new life and—even—beauty still close at hand? My mother reaches deep into the thicket of stems and blossoms, expertly feels with her eyes closed for what has died and nips it between two fingers, drawing it out, dropping it into her bag, and moves on.

*High on Everest, climbers claw at ice, gasp in the thin air, lose their footing and fall to their deaths—exposed on centuries-old glaciers that advance and splinter along the indifferent mountainside. Above twenty-five thousand feet, the human body must brutally take from itself what it needs, ignoring hunger, abandoning thought for the sake of breath. The raw calculus that drives animals in the air and the trees far below, where time's metronome beats to the intake of oxygen, becomes rashly tangled here. In the desperate last hours of ascent, climbers have been known at this altitude to pass silently the frozen corpses of comrades, stiff in the snow.*

# Thoreau's Body

Even when they stopped loving one another, and the children they had loved together turned distantly to adults, my mother and my father continued to love the same thing: the gardens that each of them planted and tended wherever they were. My parents' hopes for spring and summer stir in my own body decades after the last garden they made together was sold to strangers, even though their coming undone from one another long ago almost certainly began with their bodies—those delicate instruments of love and of loss.

My father's business was the body. Our family meals were often held up while he finished making house calls, dispensing his potions from the big leather bag that he lugged from the trunk of the car and settled every night in the same spot on the floor of my parents' bedroom closet. Their hanging clothes *whooshed* as he elbowed them aside. When my father asked his patients to undress in their homes, they took off their clothes and showed him what hurt. At home before bed, in my own dark bedroom, I offered to unbutton my pajamas so that he could fix me too, and he laughed before he kissed me goodnight.

I had my own business with doctors wearing stethoscopes like my father's, to whom my mother took me for dreaded shots and for the pink-dripped sugar cubes that freed my generation, the first in history, from fear of polio. I recognized on their office doors the two letters from which my father never loosed his grip, the magic code that he wielded: $M + D$. Those letters were printed on my father's checks, in his listing in the phone book, on the pads of stationery stacked neatly at the edge of the desk in his upstairs study. Next to the ashtray into which his overturned pipe spilled charred cherry-scented tobacco, my father kept a model of a human kidney. Two hinged plastic halves opened to blood-red tissue, revealing the molded cord of the ureter that wound between veins and arteries as smooth to my touch as toys. "Doctor Burton Jacobson," he always introduced himself, extending his title before he offered his hand.

After dinner my father would pull a chair close to the big tropical fish tank over which he presided—master of tiny bodies—in the living room. Each fish had been hand selected on one of the weekends when my father was not on call: the translucent pearl gouramis; the golden swordtails that darted in and out of plaster castles; the aquatic ferns that he had planted as carefully as his backyard garden; the ugly catfish that trolled the bottom of the tank, stirring up a cloudy mix of gray droppings and parti-colored gravel. Over the tank's side, my father hung a net for the newborn babies that the adult guppies and black mollies would otherwise eat alive. He would pull me close, reaching over my shoulder to point out the pregnant females that we needed to monitor in order to save as many of their young as we could. Sometimes my father turned off the living room lights, and the bubbling tank would hover in the room like an alien spaceship. We'd watch the neon tetras darting back and forth, leaving fluorescent streaks in the invisible water.

In the books that we read together, my father and I wondered at the miracles performed far beneath the surface of the earth and the sea, where life has learned to find its way in darkness. As cavefish have adapted to their lightless world, they've lost not only their sight but their eyes; flaps of skin have mutated over the empty orbits. At the ocean's greatest depths, nearly 90 percent of living beings manage to make their own light. Jellyfish and squid glow like X-rays, their fluid bodies outlined in eerie blue and pink, enabling them to find the mates and the prey on which the survival of their species depends. René Descartes compared the sight of luminous creatures in seawater to sparks struck off flint, and that drama—the pulsing firefly its earthly parallel, mysteriously appearing in backyards, drawing us after it hungrily with glass jars in the summer darkness— seems to this day like a kind of magic.

Sidelined during World War II by his weak eyes, my father always appears in photographs from the time he was courting my mother at college as the fellow in ordinary street clothes and thick glasses. In each glossy print bordered with tiny tanks and fighter planes and V's for *Victory*, the other girls' boyfriends pose in uniform. My father rarely spoke of the war years or of his 4-F status, of his unfitness to give his body in service to the last American war to be shared as a national mission.

In a beach photo taken just after the war, dated in the scalloped margins in blotchy blue-black fountain pen ink, my father is wearing his medical student's white coat: the uniform that he finally won. Married a year, my mother is kneeling at the apex of the photograph, between her American-born mother-in-law at ease on the Lake Michigan shore in a billowing flowered dress and her own immigrant mother clenching both fists around a dark, heavy-looking handbag as she faces into the sun. Against the washed-out sky my father's white coat glows bright. He stands slightly apart from the others, a prop on the postwar stage where this freshly forged American family is claiming its first doctor. My father's eyes remain a mysterious element in his smile, barely visible behind dense glass.

When my father's internship was completed, my parents bought a house in the suburbs, purchased seeds and power tools, gave their young bodies to the work of making a new life together. My father would brace himself with a solidly planted foot, yank the lawn mower's long cord—and the machine would roar to life, turning everything around it to silence. In its wake the disorder of growing grass was steadily tamed; flattened to the last narrow strip over which he made a single victorious pass. He'd steer the bucking engine through quivering greenness, bearing down, at once releasing a rich, sweet aroma and delivering death that we'd never know about until we found a bloodied tail among the shorn dandelion heads and the ragged fragments of clover.

My father was one of the pioneers of the contact lenses— smaller, more pliable, neatly curved over just the cornea—that were developed in the years after World War II. They amazed him with the first truly sharp correction of his vision. But the fit of mass-produced contact lenses had not yet been perfected; when a lens popped out of his eye or blew out the open window, my father would have to pull the car over to the side of the road, suddenly blinded. My parents would drop to their hands and knees, and feel in the grime around the brake pedal and the clutch for the miraculous bits of plastic.

My father had printed a single line that he loved from *Moby-Dick*, and he mounted it on the wall of his study for inspiration: "The path to my fixed purpose is laid with iron rails, whereon my soul is grooved to run." Yet—like Melville's leg-maimed Ahab—it was his own body that wrecked my father. A series of retina detachments proved impossible for his doctors to repair. First one eye went dark, and he was forced to wear a black patch over it while his vision in the other steadily dwindled, until cataract surgery granted him sight for one final year.

Then his heart weakened, that muscled chamber continuing to pump into his sixties while hoarding its secret weakness. From across the country, my father told me over the phone that the brutal bypass surgery had saved him, but I suspected that his heart was headed for disaster just the same: friendships beyond his ability to sustain, his last marriage ending in divorce, he was left alone with the one body for which medical training had not prepared him.

Finally there was cancer. I rode with him from the hospital where surgeons had removed his bladder, both of us staring out the window in awkward silence as Lake Michigan slipped by in a blur. Chained in his wheelchair to the deck of the medical taxi, my father could barely hold up his head, and he skidded helplessly back and forth each time we slowed to a stop at a red light or turned the long curves of Lake Shore Drive. I touched my father's hand, cramped fearfully over the arm of his wheelchair, but his eyes were already closed, his doomed body distant and alone.

Who are we, returning once again to the planetary surface, dropping through cloudy fluff made improbably of ice; imagining that the things we know could be forever? Below our slowly landing airplane the world seems not right, the bowl of the sky turned upside down—my mother, at home with a broken pelvis and sick lungs, a tiny star flickering in the wide dark.

My mother has long been filled with the fear of falling. She knows that when the elderly topple, the end careens suddenly closer. All around her my mother can see friends pushing walkers over the carpet, resisting distraction from every direction; neighbors taken to the hospital on stretchers who no longer return her phone calls. The old recover in this way an intimacy with the fragile beginnings of life. Like animals, they remain alert to the daily demands of survival.

My mother counts the minutes she can breathe, remains tied by the hour to the oxygen that she carries like a papoose—the baby that feeds *her*. This past winter she was back in the hospital in Chicago, coughing up blood. In New York, I tried to shut down the images clouding my mind's eye: my mother waking in the night, turning on the light to see red drenching the white tissue and staining her sticky hand. Some days she felt fine, my mother would answer when I called to ask if she was getting better; on other days she shivered as though she had a fever but her temperature remained normal. She was taking the higher dose of antibiotics that her doctor prescribed when he last saw her, but she was still dizzy. Thinking and living in days. Following the body's calendar as though that was simple.

At the end of last year's visit, my mother stood in her apartment doorway, waving goodbye as usual. She steadied herself with one hand against the door jamb, her oxygen tank backlit against the dining room strewn with newspapers and Post-it reminders, a tunnel opening like a Vermeer in her framed wake, dark volumes of furniture looming in front of windows. She told me she was slowing down, short of breath more and more, that she knew things wouldn't be getting better and I must accept that. Fingers fluttering at her mouth, blowing kisses, she looked tiny as I headed toward the elevator and then to the taxi waiting in the street, the driver taking my luggage, slamming the trunk and then the car door next to his seat, starting up the engine without knowing a thing about me or about my mother. I turned to watch the familiar streets unspool behind us—playing in reverse the film of my arrival.

Now my mother has become a wounded animal, roaring in pain, anxious about oxygen, cornered, wary of nurses' promises of improvement. "I want them to tell me what to expect, and how to handle it," she pleads with me, pulling herself up in bed so that she can meet my uncomprehending look head-on. When she first fell, she dragged herself to her feet without thinking, clinging to her walker as the front door clicked shut behind her, until the pain became too much and she crumpled again to the ground. Now she seems hollowed out, at once only her body and not at all the body that she's known. She makes her slow way to the bathroom with the help of a nurse, clenching the handles of the walker, dangling a plastic bag of used Kleenex. "I'm not myself," she turns and tells me, in tears. "I'm all broken down."

While my mother sleeps, I ride the commuter train on which I used to escape from high school, the cars plunging back into the city, north to south, following the lakeshore. The backs of the three-story apartment buildings along the way look exactly as I remember, their brick walls still scaled by frame staircases hung with laundry and flowerpots. The same gray paint seems to be fading and peeling in the prairie sun, the same barbecues and bicycles and plastic lawn chairs parked on rear porches. We pass the old landmarks—Wrigley Field and the Aragon Ballroom—and the stop where I used to get off for work at my cousin's picture-framing store in the innocent years before he died of AIDS. Auto repair shops with cracked windows still hug the edges of the tracks. At Morse Avenue, nearly the last stop before the end of the line, I can see the hand-painted signs on the immigrant-generation storefronts that already looked tired forty years ago. Through the dusty train window, time seems stubbornly stopped. But when I return to my mother's room, her body seems to be changing before my eyes, distilled down to unreachable pain.

This is what times does: remakes the world that seemed like the only world; reveals how, impossibly, that world drifts away. Illness too flings us back upon our old identities as bodies, onto ancient terrain that is at once barely remembered and deeply known. Dutch pathologists have discovered that fetal cells sometimes make their way from the uterus of a pregnant woman and implant themselves in the mother's own body. Child to mother as well as mother to child! *Microchimerism*: this counterintuitive journey is also made by other mammal species, confounding the trajectory of inheritance and our understanding of it. Chimeric, shadowy, the illusion of our separateness tugs at me like a taunt as I watch my mother's body suffer anxiously in her bed, feeling our destinies invisibly twinned, cellular.

Modern imaging plumbs the body's depths with radar, magnetism, radiation, reveals a whole world beneath the surface of the skin: the way things work, and the things that can go wrong. Yet it also reminds us that the body remains a keeper of secrets. In remission, my blood disorder is invisible even under the most powerful of microscopes. During the year when it was slowly approaching, the clues it left confused us: the filmy rainbow that I tried to blink away, blanketing my vision without warning. It would be months before we learned to read the story my eyes were trying to tell, the clumps of blood that were blocking the way to my brain. And then, scariest of all, the un-saying of *aphasia*: the scrambling of language with no explanation; words launching from my mouth like clumsy tumblers, sound blowing uselessly through the air. Even now, as I look back and remember, speech—that precious part of me—feels wounded. We like to think of illness as an anomaly, a wrong that we hope to right. Yet isn't it wellness that's the illusion, the false promise: the fragile, hovering butterfly, lightness outweighed by air, life as short as a season?

I am drinking a cappuccino in what used to be the neighborhood drugstore of my childhood, converted now into a coffee bar. From this table and chair, I can reconstruct the old geography: the shelves near the front door loaded with candy and gum, and the cashier behind them, the sound of her register taking in nickels and dimes, ringing over and over; the big freezer chest filled with popsicles and ice cream sandwiches and pint containers of rainbow sherbet puffing cold steam each time someone lifted the heavy lid. In memory this space holds still, a suspension of glass cases on which glossy yellow-and-black boxes of Jean Naté lotion and bath salts and atomizers—treasures I never saw on my mother's bedroom dresser—were buoyed like the sailboats on Lake Michigan just a few blocks away. I would stand transfixed in the slice of afternoon left at the end of the school day, watching trays of roasting salted nuts turn like a Ferris wheel, their hot, breathy scent meeting midair the thickly sweet smell of the perfume. The same black-and-white tile spreads across the floor, nicked and warped now in many spots but still the same ground on which I stood in hungry wonder more than half a century ago. Around me people I don't know read newspapers, order coffee, catch up with one another over breakfast.

What do these people see when they see me? A fattish white-haired woman in jeans and black boots, her table and her sweater littered with crumbs from the pastry she ordered with her coffee. I am still breathing, my heart pumping, my blood filling with oxygen as it used to here so many years ago. I can see the blue veins raised on the backs of my hands, feel lumpy tendons just beneath the skin—like my mother's hands, a dozen blocks away. My mother's arms are patched with raw wounds that take a long time to heal because her skin is old and thin, but just like hers my blood leaves my heart and passes under the skin's surface. Narrowing arteries squeeze past the checkpoints of organs and muscle, sustaining the rosy color of my fleshy face and my anxious tapping fingers. Yet even I cannot see the stealth passages through which disorder enters my blood, making me sick. Illness sets its own calendar, collides unexpectedly with the present with a thud—silently, secretly changes course, holds the power to make everything different.

We live in a world of disruption: migrating birds thrown fatally off course by urban lights and noise, the seas rising as glaciers melt. In Miami, salt water soaks suburban lawns, fish swim in low-lying parks. Pluto has been demoted from one of the nine planets in the solar system that we see in the nighttime sky to a large rock orbiting the sun! To be ill is, yes, to be similarly called out of the world that we count on, the reality that we take for granted. But it is also to be called more deeply into the world, to be immersed in its messiness and its movement, its ability to surprise and its mystery. Some mornings I lie in bed reluctant to open my eyes, as though that might prevent light from once again shattering against my will, from turning the world that I see into jagged pieces. I want to refuse the sick feeling of recognition that my body can go wrong without warning. The areas of the brain that control our most human functions—speech, memory, feeling—are called by neurosurgeons "eloquent"; the most essential to avoid damaging as they cut. But illness too is the body's eloquence, its own insistent language: moving, and truthful.

"How then can our harvest fail?" Thoreau called out at the triumphant completion of *Walden*'s cycle of seasons. It was on his body that Thoreau hoped to learn during those two years at the pond to register nature's miracles, intimate as the senses: to "hear the booming of the snipe; to smell the whispering sedge where . . . the mink crawls with its belly close to the ground." It bears remembering, then, that *Walden* was the work of illness, that Thoreau went to Walden Pond in illness's grieving wake.

Love and loss were the tangle that Thoreau was determined to clear at the pond, his vision of "living deliberately" and of each morning's purifying bath in Walden's water. First came the tetanus that infected his brother John's simple shaving cut—setting John's lungs into helpless spasm, leaving his locked heart drowning in fluid, his limbs contorted in Henry's useless embrace. Then what was, I believe, for Thoreau an act of love: his sorrowed body echoing the twisted grip that drew his brother into death, Thoreau nearly dying himself of a sympathetic case of lockjaw. Beloved to Thoreau as well was Ralph Emerson's son Waldo, taken at the age of five by scarlet fever.

They saw themselves as American wild boys: Thoreau embarking on his journey at Walden on July fourth, Emerson demanding "blood-warm" writing. Still, Thoreau's body would continue to unsettle him, and when the alien urge to devour a woodchuck raw suddenly took him on a twilight trail at the pond, he was silenced. Within a few years of Walden he would make his way to Mount Katahdin, pressing through uncut forests and whitewater rapids, clawing up the rubble to the mountain's fearsome summit. There—among the "gray, silent rocks," where human beings left no trace—language once more abandoned Thoreau to his own shivering flesh, his loneliness returning, once more unanswered: "I stand in awe of my body, this matter to which I am bound has become so strange to me."

On the north shore of Lake Superior, I cross a narrow bridge to the same landscape that French fur traders encountered more than three centuries ago: dense evergreens rising over rapids, their layered branches reaching toward high light. It is another July fourth, Thoreau's celebrated anniversary at Walden and a strange anniversary of my own: the date on which I was admitted to the hospital two years in a row. Unsure of my body, I keep watch over my sneakers as I cross the wet and tangled roots jamming the path into the forest, as I cling to the cliff's edge over the splendid water, the largest volume of any lake in North America. I trip on another trail winding through a series of spectacular waterfalls, come to a shocked stop face-down in the dirt, the breath knocked out of me.

"Recovery" evokes a return to equilibrium, reclaimed balance, like the return to shore of a ship that was blown off course on the high seas or the righting of a sailboat that wind brought to the brink of capsizing in wild water. In the tense moment just before a space capsule splashes down, time is suspended—until the warped vehicle with its singed patch of flag is sighted in the distance, a miracle dropping out of the clouds. Then the seconds and minutes begin to tick again.

Or does recovery contain its own limits, its own stubborn seeds of mystery, like the Iron Age bodies salvaged from centuries-old peat bogs in Denmark and Ireland, blindfolded and bandaged, inexplicably bearing signs of violence? In flight from the body's losses, Thoreau found peaceful Walden, where he rode the seasons to his own kind of clarity.

Illness is a mystery with which the body continues to haunt us. My cataracts came at exactly the same age as my father's, his legacy an old puzzle of sightlessness and isolation that I could not shake even thirty years later as I waited for surgery in yet another dull hospital corridor. I call my mother in Chicago to ask how she is feeling; when she remembers my blood and the fatigue with which illness continues to dog me, she asks the same, though her diminished hearing quickly confounds the conversation. "I love you," I try to remember to tell my mother before I hang up the phone. "Love you back," she always responds when I do.

I am drawn to beavers for their patience and their will to repair, their ability to sustain. Over and over they rebuild their dams when another animal or harsh weather takes down what they've made, breaks through the crust of mud and branches, lets water rush back in and wash out the beavers' work. The sharp teeth that the beaver uses to cut down the trees with which it builds will continue to grow as long as the beaver lives—prepared for violence, even to kill, if the beaver feels threatened.

I am body, illness tells me: a physical, working thing like the beaver, fearsome and fearful, the leavings of uncounted generations of parents and children, of their hopefulness and their disappointments. Lonely to the end, Melville reached out in an 1851 letter, alarming Nathaniel Hawthorne with his intimacy: "Whence come you, Hawthorne? By what right do you drink from my flagon of life? And when I put it to my lips—lo, they are yours and not mine." Flesh and bone, eyes and lips, hungry for woodchuck, the body can be broken, can draw us to one another, can mark the throbbing boundaries of our aloneness.

At a family funeral I watch mourners spill into daylight behind a loaded hearse, unready to release the body they loved into the grasp of death. Nor has illness readied me either to let go. Sometimes still a word floats out of my reach, leaving me wondering if it's only a balloon I've unthinkingly let go— or, instead, a sign that I'm starting to fall apart, like my father and my mother before me. Just the same, illness has made me hear freshly my own breath, intimate and necessary. "Diseases exist to remind us that we are not made of wood," Vincent van Gogh wrote in a letter from the hospital where he struggled for a final long year to recover his health. In the most famous of the paintings he made there, Van Gogh looked out through the window of the room where he slept—his body and his mind wounded—into a starry night sky that vibrated with color and emotion. The mystery of the world hovered before Van Gogh, glowing, chimeric; continued to inspire his swirling vision of beauty, the paint laid on thick as flesh.

# Book of Names

How far is it from A to B?

My mother has lived for ninety-one years, named and re-named by her mother and father and husband, logging into her address book new neighbors and nieces and nephews, penciling in their husbands and wives and children. When she remembers, she crosses out and erases the names that bad feelings and death have smudged from her lists. She asks me on a weekend visit to help her with what she can no longer manage on her own: to distill what's here into a whole; to write out clearly what remains close to her heart.

I open the book, the alphabet beginning and ending and beginning again in clumps of tangled pages. Old mimeographed lists of synagogue committees and reading groups are folded in. My sister, *ANITA*, is spelled out in block letters at the start, then my mother's friend *BATYA*, trailing a decade of moves and address changes in different ink colors. Last week Anita sent my mother, wheelchair-bound for the first time, a Rosh Hashana dinner—freshly baked challah and, in a little Tupperware container, homemade gefilte fish with sharp horseradish, her favorite—and my mother reiterates her delight when I read aloud my sister's name. "Is Batya still alive?" I push on, looking up to read my mother's face. My mother shrugs, no longer sure; they had a falling out a while ago. The minutes sag as we swerve back and forth between the first two letters of the alphabet, *A–B* on the first cardboard tab that it seems we'll never be able to turn.

It's a bit like parachuting into someone else's head, released over unfamiliar territory without a map, slowly sinking through light, aiming for distantly shadowed ground. Under *C,* for "cell phone," my mother has gathered the mobile phone numbers of all her children and grandchildren—and, on a separate line, "corned beef." Under *P* she has listed "popcorn." She's unsure how we should record the name of her accountant: under *A?* Or should we move it to *T* (for taxes) or to *I* (for income tax), or possibly *K* (for Karen). "I don't *know* Karen's last name," my mother responds, peevishly, when I ask. I can feel my own blood beating too quickly.

My mother's life has grown small in the wake of illness and injury, and she grips the pages like a wobbling anchor, as though they fix her connection to the outside world. "You'll finish this tomorrow?" she presses as I put on my coat at the end of the long day, and I don't hold back my sigh: "Unless I kill myself first!" Luckily she can't hear a lot of what I say, and I am already nodding my head, regretting my impatience.

My mother's heart is still going, but every day it gives up a little more: weakening, slowing, permitting a leak to breach its smooth-muscle wall. I press my hand on my own chest when I hear this news from my mother's doctor—hoping for a private clue from the inside. Placing an anxious finger over the vein threading in blue the soft interior of my wrist, I'm relieved to feel faint throbbing. To the far reaches of her body, my mother struggles to pump freshly red blood, to feed her ever more confused brain and the rich marrow of the bones that prevent her packed and sloshing body from collapsing like a leather sack. The heart is the world in its own way, and it telegraphs to the surface its messages and its signs, the body's strengths and weaknesses, and what it knows.

On my mental family calendar now: my mother's last Chanukah candle lighting; my mother's last Passover seder; my mother's last Yom Kippur. Shuttling back and forth between my sister's house, where the kids and their news—the acquisition of girlfriends and boyfriends and advanced degrees; career decisions, travel from continent to continent—fill the air, to my mother's room, where so much moves sluggishly, requires from me daily emotional recalibration. At Anita's house a robin's nest clings to the sunny side of the house, its delicate, impossibly blue eggs easily visible from my niece's bedroom window; in my mother's crowded room, the sound of oxygen pumping makes audible her rough pushing, breath by breath, against the limits of her body. "How was today?" I ask my mother. Time slows like her heartbeat as she strains to hear my voice through the phone and to grasp what I'm saying, and then to find an answer to this impossible question. "Okay," she finally tells me, "nothing special."

A migrating bird reads the magnetic fields of the earth like a compass: creating its own internal map, marking its route to where it needs to go in order to survive the changing seasons. Thrown off course by experimenting scientists, birds will right themselves midair, bank sharply over water or land, then recover their original path toward home. The heart of the ruby-throated hummingbird takes up nearly 2.5 percent of its total body weight—five times the relative size of the human heart—enabling it to beat over one thousand times per minute, powering flight nine hundred miles across the Gulf of Mexico and the Caribbean. But that kind of energy can only last about five years. My mother can no longer remember the names of the neighbors and the family members filling her address book, can no longer walk to breakfast without becoming winded. I ask her if she is frightened. No, she tells me, she accepts what is ahead, but to feel her life steadily shrink is, she says, "dis-heartening."

When Moses's brother, Aaron, struck the water with his staff, the great Nile and the other rivers of Pharaoh's kingdom were turned to blood, leaving fish suddenly swimming in redness and dying in it, imposing throughout the land an unquenchable thirst. At the Passover seder, we spill blood again, dipping our fingertips into sticky, sweet wine, sinking flesh into symbol, sounding aloud the ten warning plagues. Blood's alarming peal, the Hebrew word *dom*, intoned; then the insects and the infections and the darkness. And the final horror, the slaying of the firstborn, meant to break Pharaoh—and to break his people's hearts.

My mother's doctor holds her stethoscope against my mother's blouse, closing her eyes to hear everything she can, then opening them to meet my mother's anxious look. My mother's body has logged millions of heartbeats: pounded life through her veins when she competed in citywide ball games as a kid; when she called down the block for her own children to come home for the dinner that she'd cooked; when she dug gardens and harvested what she had grown in them; when she bicycled Chicago's lakeside parks and played tennis doubles and joined in folk dancing on a ship's deck headed down the Volga toward Saint Petersburg. But what, really, can her heart say now? My mother can no longer manage all the buttons and zippers to dress herself; is no longer able to find her underpants, their nylon worn to a silky smoothness thinner than skin, or her socks. Her doctor tries to explain that if my mother's deep cough doesn't resolve in another day she will have to send her to the hospital. "Because I can't take care of myself?" my mother blurts out, afraid and ashamed; her doctor emphatically shakes her head, "No, no, that's not why." My mother shuts her eyes tight to still the world's dizziness.

"*Kol Nidre* commands the acknowledgment of time," the rabbi introduces Yom Kippur's initial prayer, announcing the most sacred hours—sunset to sunset—on the Jewish calendar. In my mother's room, I've set up her TV so we can watch together as the service is streamed live from Manhattan to Chicago. My mother raises her head from her chest and hums softly as a cello begins to play on-screen. In more than ninety years of living, how many times has my mother listened to the aching chant that follows, salvaging what she can from time's rawness?

At this season of the year we look back, and then forward: hoping for signs, trying to accept the fact of change ahead that we cannot know. *Who will live and who will die? Who in their time, and who not their time? Who by fire and who by water?* The ancient poem provokes us as we recite it, placing before us the inevitability of hurt. This year I feel a tug at my throat, feel my mother struggling for breath, as I join her and the voices of the televised congregation: *Who by strangling and who by stoning?*

I toss the pages of my mother's old address book into the trash, letter by letter. "She's gone," my mother tells me. Or: "Don't bother. I'll never call her again." Sometimes my mother pauses to ask, using the name that she gave to me, "Do you remember her, Joanne? Do you remember going to their house in California?" Hours pass in the small room, the heat turned up so that my mother won't become chilled, the walls closing in as the same names appear over and over because my mother has listed them again and again rather than searching for what she needs among the tangled alphabets. My mother's Book of Life: *Muriel Levy, Lorna Mae Israel*—each name accumulating new addresses and phone numbers, trailing the scratched-out names of husbands. I continue, no longer resisting what she is asking of me. At the very edge of loss and of mystery, my mother pauses to catch her breath, and we take turns calling out the names, letting go one by one.

# Acknowledgments

Completing work that skates this close to life—to breath and to blood—depends on love and on community, and I have been lucky to have both.

Thanking my mother, Florence Jacobson, is bittersweet, as I so wish that she had lived to see this book in print. She was without question a reluctant subject but, equally and unfailingly, a model of generosity and spirit and decency. My sister, Anita Jacobson, and brother-in-law Eddie Feldman have been allies and partners to me over these years of writing.

At Yeshiva University, Karen Bacon, Selma Botman, Barry Eichler, and Morton Lowengrub provided funding and time to complete these essays. And Fred Sugarman, my beloved intellectual pal, has shared so much of my work.

My writing colleagues at YU—Barbara Blatner, Paula Geyh, Joan Haahr, Johanna Lane, and Liesl Schwabe—have taken the time to be readers and to encourage me. At a crucial moment, Lauren Fitzgerald extended to me a hand of support and kindness that I will never forget. And my writing has benefited from the counsel and encouragement, elsewhere, of

William Merrill Decker, Elizabeth Grubgeld, Natania Rosenfeld, and Katie Watson.

For precious, decades-long mentorship and friendship as fundamental as sustaining my idea of myself as a writer, I am grateful to Richard McCann and to Stephen Donadio: *family*. I am grateful to my rabbi, Sharon Kleinbaum, for helping me to incorporate illness—and gratitude—into my life: *tov l'hodot*. And I am grateful to David Sugarman, who emerged magically at just the right time as a partner in my writing life.

Thank you to the Ragdale Foundation, the Virginia Center for the Creative Arts, and the Anderson Center for providing quiet, time, and supportive companions.

For healing when my life depended on it, and for wisdom and compassion, I thank Elizabeth Belkin, Carol Diamond, and Kevin Troy.

So many other friends and neighbors and family members have supported me and the completion of this work in so many ways—from making daily phone calls to making chicken soup; from staying close to cat sitting. I thank all of them, particularly Barbara Dolgin, Hanna Gafni, and Diane Pearl. And to Tahl Mayer and Ali Shrago-Spechler: thank you for giving your big hearts to love and to art, especially in such dark times!

At The University of Utah Press, I feel extraordinarily lucky to have benefited from Janalyn Guo's support and patience, as well as the attentive, helpful critiques of Scott Abbott and Jennifer Sinor. And I thank Nikki Bazar for her sensitive editing.

I am grateful most of all to my partner and wife, Ellen Wertheim. She has lived every minute and every word of this work with me, in sickness and in health. May that partnership in love and creativity continue to sustain both of us—with every last breath.